SURVIVING
COMPASSION FATIGUE

Additional Acclaim for *Surviving Compassion Fatigue*:

Beverly Kyer has written a book of healing for those not only in the healing professions but relevant to all human "Beverly D. Kyer's powerful book provides much needed information to support caregivers. In reading her book; I discovered so many of us are impacted by compassion fatigue. In the sharing of her personal story, important caregiver statistics, the wisdom and practical steps she brings awareness and support to our caregivers in needed and powerful ways. She speaks so powerfully to making sure we are caring for the caregivers....beginning with caregivers discovering how to take care of themselves first so that they aren't serving from a place of depletion. This book is a valuable resource for caregivers and I believe a for all of us to develop a better understanding of compassion fatigue. Compassion fatigue, I believe, will either effect you directly, or someone you know. The more informed and empowered we become, the healthier, more balanced, vibrant, our lives and those of caregivers (on those they support) will be.

- Rebecca Hall Gruyter, Women's Empowerment Leader

Beverly Kyer has written a book of healing for those not only in the healing professions but relevant to all human services workers...not merely social workers, but teachers, police officers, firefighters, ministers, and administrators. Surviving Compassion Fatigue should be a required course for all undergraduate and graduate level students entering into human services work and this book should provide the framework.

- Bryan Post, CEO www.postinstitute.com

SURVIVING
COMPASSION FATIGUE

Help for Those Who Help Others

The Story, the Mission and a Gift
From a Compassion Fatigue Survivor

BY BEVERLY D. KYER, MSW, CSW, ACSW
FOREWORD BY DR. RICHARDS P. LYON

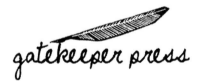

gatekeeper press

Published by Gatekeeper Press
3971 Hoover Rd. Suite 77
Columbus, OH 43123-2839

Layout Design by: Mr. Merwin D. Loquias

ISBN: 9781619844902
eISBN: 9781619844919

Printed in the United States of America

To God, who is my source, and for my life, assignment, and gifts for this mission.
And to my children, Michael, Melvina, and Jamal for being my pride and inspiration

We delight in the beauty of the butterfly, but rarely admit the changes it has gone through to achieve that beauty.

–Maya Angelou

CONTENTS

ACKNOWLEDGEMENTS

My Gratitude goes to the following:

My family in California, Florida, France, Georgia, New Jersey and New York City

Dr. Richards Lyon who always endeavored to ease my stress every time I brought my child to him for care. Thank you for your totally loving and compassionate care

Bishop Carl C. Smith for leading me to embrace the "Covenant Promises"

My Publisher Cy Forh and Editor Jonathan Williams for believing in my work

My Cardiologist who wishes anonymity; who made the right diagnosis.

Peter Challenor, my Acupuncturist and Dr. Robert Woodbine, the healing voice from across the country, whose wisdom and skill aided and sustained me on my journey to wellness

My neighbor Joanne, who drove me to cardiac rehab

The courageous contributors who shared their stories:

Brian Post for introducing me to the construct called compassion fatigue

John Prindle, whose book inspired me to finish writing mine

Loral Langemeier for teaching me entrepreneurial practices

Sylvia High for helping me to discover and move through the blind spots to achieve my goals

John Robinson who shared knowledge to finish this book

Vicki Ward for her very generous mentoring on self-publishing

Bob Friend, my former Supervisor who developed and nurtured my knowledge of the Child Welfare System

Jakki Koslow, Sylvia Pizzini and Morgen Hume for invaluable linkages to resources and data from The Child Welfare system

The great folks at Steeltown Café in Pittsburg CA. for the perfect atmosphere and customer service for a writer

To my neighbor Michelle who has a sharp eye for grammar and context

FOREWORD

I am thrilled that Beverly should believe I share her views. As a pediatric urologist, I have enjoyed her faith and friendship for all of the years as we have worked with her son Jamal, who carries on his mother's intents and wisdom in this ever-changing world.

A caregiver is a relatively new profession, although it has been a no name practice for centuries. It is now more demanding as we live longer, but pay the ever more demanding price of war's creation, seeming never to diminish.

The caregiver is just as much at risk as a young battle fatigue survivor. The caregiver, too, must order his or her life to make for continued effectiveness. Beverly is among the first to recognize this, as she translates her own life threatening experiences into a gospel of positive thinking and acting. Her story is likely to be a classic as she includes seminal works of others, hoping to make the story and lessons complete. Thank you, Beverly.

Sunday, September 14th, 2014
Richards Lyon, M.D. (Dr. Dick)
Napa, California

INTRODUCTION

This book is for all professional service providers, caregivers, and helpers who struggle to restore and recharge their mind, body, and spirit as they meet the needs of their clients. Often, as caregivers attempt to help their clients deal with their losses, pain, and struggles, many end up taking on the negative emotions and pain of their clients. This is often compounded by the strain of working under persistent pressure, often with limited resources and a reduced staff.

This book will provide you with strategies and techniques to protect yourself from becoming emotionally overwhelmed by your work. My objective is to help you retrain your thought patterns to increase your self-regulation and internal calm and decrease stress, all while increasing your effectiveness and motivation even under distressing, frustrating, and threatening circumstances.

DISCLAIMER

This book has several theories. Some of them are well known and evidence-based, and some are new and cutting-edge. However, theories are just that, theories. This book is rich with my opinions, the opinions of others who have labored along side me, and the opinions of those who have preceded me in this field of study. When I lecture around the country, I always encourage my audiences to think critically, seek answers, and decide what works best for them. I encourage you to do the same.

Further, compassion fatigue can result in serious and even life-threatening consequences when the service provider does not attend to their own self-care. I am neither a medical doctor nor a licensed psychologist; therefore, my recommendations in this book are not to replace sound medical and psychological evaluation and treatment. In fact, I always urge my audiences to be more diligent about routine checkups so that they can detect health problems as early as possible, thus allowing early intervention so that a minor concern does not become a major crisis.

CHAPTER 1:
EMPATHY, OR WHY WE DO
WHAT WE DO

If it's not working, make it work.

—My father

Before we move forward to talk about and explore compassion fatigue—what it is, how it affects us, and how we heal from it—it might be good to look back and remind ourselves why we started working as a service provider in the caring professions in the first place. It will be important to remember why we do what we do as we go forward and talk about and attempt to counter the effects of compassion fatigue.

EMPATHY IS NOT UNIVERSAL

During my 35-year career as a social worker, I have worked in federal, county, and private organizations where I have had the honor of working alongside staff from multiple backgrounds and in multiple work settings, including collateral work with state workers in cities across the US. One of the many lessons I learned during my varied work experiences was that empathy is not a quality possessed by all men and women. For many, empathy must be cultivated. In many of the trainings I do on trauma and grief and loss impacts, whether the impacts be on children, youth or adults, I have had to include exercises to promote empathy for many in my audience. It seems when people have not experienced or been directly exposed to tragic and painful situations themselves, they have difficulty understanding why all people do not simply recover quickly and move on to bigger and better successes. They have a hard time understanding why recovery from trauma requires so much time. To them, the time and effort don't seem necessary and don't make sense.

Even people who have experienced and recovered from tragedies in their own lives may be unable to realize that other emotional, developmental, or environmental factors exist that affect others but do not affect them. It is these factors that make it more difficult for some to be able to rebound as quickly and successfully as them. My exercises are intended to expose and sensitize many to these factors, factors which may overwhelm the capacity of traumatized and victimized persons to recover in a timely manner.

Of course, there are those who live in environments where they are completely shielded from the misfortunes of others. And then there are those who choose to avoid acknowledging unpleasant circumstances faced by others. These few are the people who often blame the victim for being a victim.

UNDERSTANDING BREEDS EMPATHY AND REALISTIC EXPECTATIONS

I believe that the key to having empathy is having knowledge and insight of the vast complexities that exists within each individual. This can include not only what the struggling individual knows (or does not know), but also what they are able to believe, perceive, access, and act on. It can also include awareness of the information sources an individual uses as well as their level of fear or courage. And don't forget that each person has heard different messages as they grew up and has a different capacity to change and grow. And lastly, not everyone has the same support network, nor are they able to accept and deal with support equally when it is offered to them.

Asking the right questions to uncover these complexities requires curiosity and serves two key purposes. First, it eliminates prejudgment and expands our understanding while it opens the pathway to helping a struggling client or patient. Second, regarding our own self-care, having a deeper understanding of the human condition can eliminate much frustration and sleepless nights as we view the people we help through a larger lens and set reasonable expectations for their progress and for our effectiveness.

THE EPIDEMIC OF A LACK OF EMPATHY

After each State of the Union address by our President, I listen to just a portion of rebuttal, which is delivered by a member of the opposing political party. Obviously, the rebuttal usually speaks to a very different viewpoint about the needs and nature of our country and its citizens. During one rebuttal I recall, the person started off sharing a story about an earlier time in their life when they were faced with challenges and worked hard to overcome these challenges. Next, this person spoke about the many jobs and tasks they performed to reach the level of success they live in today. On first hearing, one might get the impression that this person was speaking to the working class, trying to establish a shared commonality, one where we are all part of the American experience.

They seemed to be saying, "I had to roll up my sleeves and dig deep just as you have." But I don't think that this was their message. Instead, I believe their message was "I got to where I am because I had to perform various tasks and work very hard, and you should be able to do the same." Because the speaker assumed that everyone should easily be able to do as they had done and with no excuses, I think that the rebuttal speaker was a perfect example of someone lacking in knowledge, insight, and awareness of the complexities of the human capacity and the human condition. They spoke as someone lacking in empathy.

I like reading some biographies and watching documentaries about great humanitarians and so many of them I have come to realize have experienced significant or grave difficulties in their own past histories. Or, at least they have borne witness to the sufferings of others. I am convinced that for many of them and certainly in my own earlier life experiences and exposures to losses and tragedies that it has been my journey through these dark areas in life that prepared and equipped me to serve and be a hand up for others who are struggling. When I see a man, woman or child trying to climb out of a hole, or sliding down into one, I can grasp so clearly many other factors that may be impeding their desire and capacity to improve their own circumstances without empathic help, support and resources. This level of understanding; this quality of empathy has helped me tremendously to approach difficult scenarios with people in need with a much greater inner calm and peace.

EMPATHY IS REQUIRED FOR OUR CALLING

I have found that most of us who have been called to work in the fields of child welfare, adult protection, and rescue services, for instance, "get it." We can see beyond our own life experiences and have empathy for the trials and traumas of others. I feel that many in the helping professions possess this quality of empathy.

Empathy, however, can be a double-edged sword. On one hand, having it can reduce some of the frustration and feelings of sadness and being overwhelmed inherent in human service work. On the other hand, it can expose us to these very same emotions. We need to strike a balance in how we chose to think, because what we believe about another person's struggles can help determine our own internal dialog and ultimately our level of inner peace (or lack thereof).

Child trauma specialist Dr. Bruce Perry has stated many times that the service we do can be emotionally taxing and can wear our bodies out. We have, or have met coworkers who have, thrown up a protective shield to ward off emotional exhaustion that can result from work-related stress, which can include client rage, client death, overly heavy caseloads, reduced staffing and resources, etc.

When this occurs, we sometimes depersonalize or dehumanize our clients. Again, we mostly do this to protect ourselves rather than because we lack humanity. This depersonalization often has two consequences which only further increase the negative aspects of the work we do. First, when our clients notice our depersonalization or absence of empathy, they often become distrustful and shut down their communication, therein limiting or shutting off their own effective treatment or care.

Second, our clients lock in their pre-existing negative material that needs to be dealt with. Ultimately, any chance of a working relationship between client and caregiver is aborted, which stops any healing, growth, or progress. The client is not helped, and the worker feels increasingly frustrated and fatigued.

One of the agencies I worked at for a number of years incorporated a practice they called "asking curious questions" as part of their staff orientations and ongoing supervisory and staff development. This meant respectfully asking questions in a non-interrogating tone and manner, such as: "Can you tell me more about that? How has that worked for you in the past? What comes up for you when this happens? What do you want to see happen in these situations? How did you hope he (or she) would respond back to you?" And so on.

By being curious, in a respectful way, of a struggling client's needs, the client is able to give you more of their story, which can give you greater understanding of their suffering and struggle. We can then see a much bigger picture that includes multiple elements and factors, rather than a narrow viewpoint that often comes from trying to communicate with a resistant or non-compliant client.

At the same time, we need to keep our expectations reasonable and not assume full burden for others' suffering or problem resolution. We are responsible for the quality of the effort we give to every situation, but not for the outcome. What we get to give our clients always is "the experience of us," which is a different experience than they have had before. This experience of us includes the respect we give, our attention, our willingness to listen, our caring, and our support and resources. To make this happen, I recommend changing in the language we use going into the work relationship, by shifting from "I will" to "we will" as we work through problems together with our clients.

MY MISSION

My mission in life and with this book is to share what it was like before and after I learned to take care of myself, to warn others of the potential dangers of inadequate self-care, and to help others see alternatives to the way we as helpers live our lives. I want to teach others how to employ intentional self-care and self-regulation strategies and to make our wellbeing a top priority so that we can remain vital and available to help those in need. My mission is to help you recharge your mind, body, and spirit.

In this book, I will try to define compassion fatigue and alert you to its warning signs, symptoms, and impacts. I will also provide strategies, interventions and tools for avoiding it and managing it in your life. My hope is that this book will help you to know what you need to do that is in your best interest. I especially want you to know that you have the power to restore and maintain your own health and wellbeing throughout your dedicated and compassionate service years to others.

CHAPTER 2:
MY STORY

We cannot, in a moment, get rid of habits of a lifetime.

–Mahatma Ghandi

It was the morning of January 5th 2002, and I felt the gentle sunlight as it kissed me awake. I hate being jarred awake by an alarm clock and only use one if I have an early morning flight, preferring instead to leave my shutters open after I turn off the lights so that I am eased into a new day by the softly rising sunlight.

However, as I awoke on this morning, I heard a strange noise. Someone was crumpling a paper bag in my room. I couldn't remember if my adult son was in the house, as he was frequently on business travel. But I realized that even if he was, he would not enter my bedroom without knocking first. My next thought was of an intruder in my bedroom, so I played possum.

As I lay still I tried to sense the intruder's location. My master bedroom is large with a reading area and small library and walking space, so there were a few spots in my room where an intruder could be at a distance from my bed, but judging by the crumpling noise, this person was close. But if they were there, I couldn't see them. So staying still, I eased my eyes open and scanned my room.

No one was there!

I lay there for a short while, nervous and perplexed, when I realized that the strange crumpling sound was coming from me. It was my own breathing. As I hoisted myself up on my elbows I felt a great pressure in my chest in sync with each breath I took. Startled, I then realized that I was all alone in my house and apparently quite sick. With some difficulty, I eased my legs over the side of the bed, made it across the room to my reading recliner, and sat down and dialed my doctor.

I soon learned that I had just survived a flare-up of restrictive cardio myopia. This is a heart chamber muscle disease that impedes the pumping of blood in and out of the heart, reducing the flow of oxygen rich blood to the brain and body, resulting in a debilitating fatigue. In me it also caused a flooding in my lungs and was the reason I needed to sit upright in a chair day and night to sleep; otherwise, I felt like a bear was sitting on my chest and I could not breathe because my lungs were filling up with fluid.

There was no one single incident that added up to create my fatigue. But if I had to point to one trigger event, it seems that the 9/11 tragedy was the proverbial straw that broke the camel's back. Over the months following 9/11, years of stored tragedies and sadness began to seep out as memory after memory came spilling out at unpredictable and unprovoked times. I could now no longer shove these memories and feelings back in, sealing them over as I had done so many times before. Now, I would see faces of the children that suffered and struggled and the many that had died at the Pediatric Oncology Center during my first job as a Social Worker. My compassion fatigue had begun, and unpleasant memories began to plague me.

I remembered the children's' cries and their parents' grief. Images of the fear and confusion and hopelessness in the children's' eyes as they went through frightening and painful procedures assailed me.

I remembered hugging a little boy just moments before he died. His body was so emaciated that I could feel the bones under his skin. I took care to be very gentle in my embrace for I feared by hugging him too tightly the bones would tear through his fragile, thin skin. I also remembered how his breath smelled of Carnation milk.

I remembered a girl whose mother had lost her way to hard-core drugs, who had repeatedly failed multiple attempts at rehabilitation. During her struggles, she had often left her children vulnerable. The dashed hopes and deep grief that her children bore were palpable when I would meet with them.

I remembered countless Vietnam veterans, their spirits broken by the atrocities they experienced. Some spewed rage, some stayed drunk, many became homeless, and some ended their lives.

I remembered the boy who saw his father shoot his mother to death, his mixture of rage, sorrow, and guilt pouring out because he could not save his mother, even though he had begged her many times to run away.

I remembered the mother whose life disintegrated after the rape and homicide of her daughter on a college campus. I learned later that the mother committed suicide over guilt she felt about (reluctantly) agreeing to send her daughter to that college to live in a dormitory.

I remembered the children who were raped and beaten.

And I remembered the boy in foster care who was murdered, in a case of mistaken identity, while walking home from school one day.

I remembered too many events and scenarios to mention them all. My point is, that by keeping so much pain buried deep inside, shunning opportunities to process my personal experiences, I was now experiencing a tidal wave of unpleasant thoughts and traumatic images that had almost taken control of my life. I failed to process these triggers, being too busy focusing on the multitude of needs facing me every day.

This deep well of feelings and emotions would not be ignored. I began to express angry emotions which were uncharacteristic of me. I would see coworkers babbling on about some concern and get annoyed or impatient with them, which often led me to argue with them over something insignificant. I also wanted to avoid parents of foster children who seemed to be blocking their child's progress regarding child safety or a much-needed intervention.

My sleep began to suffer as well. I often could not sleep, staying awake until the early hours of the morning. On top of that, when I did sleep I often experienced sleep disturbances and nightmares and would wake up sweating and crying or even screaming. I would use those sleepless nights to catch up on documentation, the only thing I could do to fill the time until morning. But when I finished typing, I would close my eyes and again see injured children.

My eating habits were no better. Most of my meals were on the run: gas station honey coated nuts, biscuits, potato chips, and soda or coffee. And I ate a lot of white flour products, which seemed to keep me going almost like a stimulant.

And of course, my workplace had other issues that contributed to my stress. Our department experienced the loss of a wonderful Director and Supervisor. There were unstable shifts in the focus and infra-structure of our work environment during the long wait for their replacement, and we lacked clarity about our mission and operating procedures. Some of our former collegial work relationships began to fray; some became toxic. Our program also suffered from declining resources, adding to acute regret I felt when I could not provide for the needs of my clients.

But did I stop and get help? Hardly. When my life gets very difficult, instead of sitting down, resting, and really taking stock, I mobilize at a very high level. Up to now, my ability to work hard and mobilize had usually been a good thing. Actually, I am one of the more reliable persons on my team because I take urgent and persistent action in the face of difficulty. I was driven in part by a message my father had given to my sister and I: "If things are not working, make it work." He worked hard and practiced what he preached and died of heart failure when he was only 66.

Not surprisingly, my principle hero and model was my father. My father was a remarkable man and was the person who inspired me the most. He worked nights full time for the railroad, and during the day he was a commercial sign painter/entrepreneur; he also managed multiple church duties as a Deacon and Trustee. Daddy took care of household chores frequently as my mother was often ill. He never missed any of our school events, recitals, concerts, or sports activities, and he took us everywhere he could think of to expand our social, moral, and cultural development.

My father, and mother, alternately walked my sister and me to school. Often, I would look up from work at my school desk and see my father peeking through the window of the door to my classroom. All the other students usually saw him too. Needless to say, I was one of the best behaved children in school.

My father moved through these activities quickly, efficiently, calmly, and with absolute intent. He was amazing. We could always depend on my father to show up and deliver. I adored him and I determined to be just like him.

At this point, you are probably wondering when my father slept. On rare occasions, my father would sleep in the daytime after he walked my sister and I to school, but only when he had no other commitment that day. More often, he slept about four hours after dinner was finished, and then he was up and off to work at the railroad for the 11 pm shift. His goal in life seemed to be to never let his family down, and he didn't. I too embraced his goal of always being dependable, both for my own children, as well as for those to whom I provided direct care and compassionate service.

Besides being my father's daughter, as they say, other factors contributed to the way I worked and lived. From both the maternal and paternal side of my family, I was given the deeply rooted southern custom of taking care of your neighbors. I observed and modeled my parents, grandparents, and extended family members who demonstrated great compassion and effort for all people, especially any person or family who was struggling. I adored my family, and I am proud to be one of them, some of whom are my heroes. As such, I selected my careers, first, Elementary Education, and later, Clinical Social Work based on the way I was raised. In my mind, these careers gave me the greatest opportunity to be of service to people. To me this was God's work.

My empathic understanding of the pain and struggles of others and my determination to help, combined with many years of stored in unprocessed sadness made me a great empath; just the kind of social worker that people could trust, talk to, and count on. I should have learned early on how to practice self-care. But I didn't.

I had no life outside of work, but I didn't know it. Helper had become my entire identity. I found no pleasure even in conference trips to beautiful places like Scottsdale and Seattle. I would fly in, do the work I had come to do, sleep little, work some more, and then fly home without taking any time to enjoy the surroundings. I actually had some time to enjoy some of the sites and activities; I simply had no interest. I was oblivious to my exhaustion. Instead, I pushed through relying on a combination of adrenalin and love. I was like a prize fighter getting up from the mat in the ring, dazed and somewhat unstable in my footing, making my way back into the battle for the next set of blows because I wouldn't listen to my inner voicing pleading with me to stay down.

Not surprisingly, my body got more and more taxed, and more and more I started to lose control of my emotions. There were times throughout the day when my nerves got so intense, so raw that I would shake uncontrollably. And then it happened.

I was upstairs alone in the office working one day when the intrusive thoughts again overtook me. I felt at once sad and angry and at the same time anxious to be productive. But my body was shaking so uncontrollably that I had to try to calm myself. I paced back and forth in my office, hoping to walk off the discomfort but it only became more intense. I then started pumping my hands and arms up and down first on the desk and then in the air, as if this would help me regain control of myself. Had someone witnessed this, they might have thought I was throwing a tantrum. I feared I was losing my mind and about to have a nervous breakdown. But the more I tried to stem the flood of emotions and my shaking, the worse I felt. All at once, a feeling inside of my stomach and my throat arose and out came little moans, and then I noticed that I was screaming. Horrified that someone would hear (fortunately no one else was on the second floor at that time) and put me in a straitjacket, I still could not stop screaming. The screams were a release that soon evolved into wrenching waves of crying. I cried and cried until I was spent and fell asleep at my desk.

It wasn't until one of my doctors, an internist, diagnosed my two cardiac episodes (particularly the second one, which landed me in rehab) as "broken heart syndrome," that I realized that my health episodes happened not long after traumatic events, like the shooting death of two of the high schoolers I worked with.

Because I was doing service for others, I made what I believe is a common mistake. I failed to count the cost of the nature of the work which had multiple crises driven and tragic circumstances, and the time expended to meet an ever increasing flood of deadlines, emergencies and daily commitments. I failed to take time for myself for rest and restoration. My focus was totally on the needs of others and the care I could give to them. I totally disregarded and overlooked the care I needed to also give to myself.

The moral of my story is that I did not collapse because of the work. My cardio issues and compassion fatigue happened because I did not care for myself. Again, despite being a professional caregiver, I had neglected my own self-care. Had I taken time to process and integrate those experiences, I might not have held on to so many years of stored sorrowful content. But I didn't. And so it all came to a head that morning in my bedroom.

CHAPTER 3:
WHAT IS COMPASSION FATIGUE?

Knowledge is power.

—Sir Francis Bacon

So what exactly is compassion fatigue? This brief chapter will hopefully give you a better idea of what it is, and what it isn't.

A SIMPLE DEFINITION

Compassion fatigue is a syndrome which consists of various symptoms that mirror post-traumatic stress disorder (PTSD) and is the suffering and secondary trauma experienced by a caregiver or service worker who deals with people who are the victims of trauma. While the caregiver or service worker did not experience the trauma firsthand, they experience a secondary trauma from treating or dealing with someone who has experienced firsthand trauma. According to the Oxford English Dictionary (OED), compassion fatigue was added as a new term in draft additions as recently as 2002.

HISTORY OF COMPASSION FATIGUE

Before going further, let's talk briefly about the history of the term compassion fatigue. To begin with, compassion fatigue is nothing new. According to Dr. Charles Figley, a world-renown authority of compassion fatigue, the study of human reactions to traumatic events can be traced to the earliest medical writings in Kunus Pyprus, written around 1900 B.C. in Egypt (Figley, 1995).

The recent (circa 1980s) emergence of this field resulted from a growing awareness of the long-term impacts of shocking events. The American psychiatric Association's third edition of the Diagnostic and Statistical Manual of Mental Disorders [DSM – III]" in 1980, recognized post-traumatic stress disorder as a legitimate psychiatric disorder that can be accurately diagnosed and treated. The APA modified criteria for symptoms in their 1994 edition, and these criteria became popular with many service providers who work directly with traumatized people. While few studies reported on people indirectly or secondarily impacted, literature on burnout and countertransference pointed to the vulnerability of the service providers and caregivers who experience similar stress from their jobs.

An early use of the term was in a 1981 US document on immigration policy. In the early 1990s the news media in the United States incorrectly used the term to describe the public's lack of patience, or perhaps simply the editors' lack of patience, with "the homeless problem," which had previously been presented as an anomaly or even a "crisis" which had only existed for a short time and could presumably be solved somehow. The term was also used in 1992 when Carla Johnson used the term in a nursing magazine to describe nurses who deal with hospital emergencies. Compassion fatigue has been studied by the field of traumatology, where it has been called the "cost of caring" for people facing emotional pain.

Compassion fatigue has also been called "secondary victimization" (Figley, 1982), "secondary traumatic stress" (Figley, 1983, 1985, 1989; Stamm, 1995; 1997), "vicarious traumatization" (McCann & Pearlman, 1989; Pearlman & Saakvitne, 1995), and "secondary survivor" (Remer and Elliott, 1988a; 1988b). Other related conditions are "rape-related family crisis" (Erickson, 1989; White & Rollins, 1981), and "proximity" effects on female partners of war veterans (Verbosky and Ryan, 1988). Compassion fatigue has been called a form of burnout in some literature. However, unlike compassion fatigue, burnout is related to chronic tedium in careers and the workplace, rather than exposure to specific kinds of client problems such as trauma.

Academic literature often uses the more technical term secondary traumatic stress disorder in place of compassion fatigue. The term "compassion fatigue" is considered by some to be somewhat euphemistic.

One measure of compassion fatigue is in the ProQOL, or Professional Quality of Life Scale. Another is the "Secondary Traumatic Stress Scale" ("Compassion Fatigue," 2015. Retrieved from http://en.wikipedia.org/w/index.php?title=Compassion_fatigue &oldid=639625141 Last visited Feb. 16, 2015).

As the Compassion Fatigue Awareness Project states, when caregivers, who have a strong identification with those suffering, fail to practice self-care they can be prone to destructive behaviors.

COMPASSION FATIGUE AND PTSD

To go a little deeper, let's take a closer look at compassion fatigue by defining PTSD, which is mentioned in the definition I quoted at the beginning of this chapter. PTSD is a disorder that affects people who have experienced extreme traumatic or violent events in their lives. This can include people who have experienced natural or man-made disasters as well as people who are victims of violent crimes, domestic violence, and sexual or physical abuse. Not only do the symptoms of compassion fatigue often resemble those of PTSD, but as a helper, you are often impacted by those who suffer from PTSD, which is why it's important to know better what PTSD is.

So, compassion fatigue is a potentially devastating syndrome that impacts people physically, mentally and emotionally and results from absorbing and internalizing the emotions, pain and suffering of others. In your work or studies you also may have heard the terms "secondary traumatic stress" or "vicarious trauma." Both of these are more clinical terms used to describe compassion fatigue, and I will be using them as well. Thus, this secondary trauma can affect people who provide services, care, and support to any of the following: victims of direct traumatic experiences, those who suffer from emotional, mental or physical illnesses, and those who are experiencing acute and chronic distress.

Because compassion fatigue can result from vicariously experiencing a psychic injury and/or a life threatening event in the lives of others, it's not surprising that people who develop compassion fatigue report episodes of fear, depression, confusion, helplessness, hopelessness, feeling out of control, extreme mood swings, avoidance behaviors, etc., which are often the very symptoms that those who suffer from PTSD also experience (Figley, 1995).

EXAMPLES OF COMPASSION FATIGUE

Think of the police and first responders at a school shooting who are tasked with recovering the bodies of children who had been shot multiple times. Now let's suppose that one or more of these first responders on their first day of duty or are returning from a restful vacation. Any symptoms they now display are not the result of being burned out. Instead, they are experiencing secondary trauma caused by the trauma they have just witnessed.

Let's also consider the grief counselors and therapists who console grieving parents, classmates, and teachers who survived the shooting. These helpers are secondarily traumatized by the images, sounds (screams and crying), the smells and suffering they witness. Like the police and EMTs who are assisting, these helpers will remember forever the experiences and the trauma they have beheld, memories which will likely resurface with intensity each time they read or hear about similar tragedies.

And let's not forget the police, probation and parole officers who are tasked day to day with viewing and interviewing the victims, survivors, and perpetrators of these types of crimes. These personnel must evaluate the circumstances, write reports, and work directly with perpetrators. These too are also at risk for experiencing compassion fatigue by experiencing this secondary trauma.

And last but not least, are the various medical personnel who work rapidly to provide triage and emergency care in an intense battle to save lives. Often in spite of their diligent efforts, they too bear witness to suffering and loss of life as well as the grief of surviving relatives and friends.

I often do debriefing sessions with social workers, therapists, medical personal, teachers, and the various staff who make up crisis response teams. These sessions are often in response to a tragedy experienced by children and/or adults, with the great majority of these sessions directly related to death. The sorrow in the room is heavy with the question "why" and how such a thing could happen and especially to the vulnerable and innocent. Compassionate people feel deep sorrow about the loss of life. In cases where they may have known the victim, they remember better days and feel the lost hope for a future that will never happen. Often, those who deal with the disaster wish that it could've been prevented, because most people with this level of humanity feel a keen sense of responsibility for all of humanity.

WHAT COMPASSION FATIGUE ISN'T

Let's talk briefly about what compassion fatigue isn't. In previous years, "burnout" has been the focus for diminished capacity, diminishing quality of service, and low productivity in the helping professions and caregiving roles. Burnout, which is a component of compassion fatigue, is the stress which results from overwhelming work demands. These demands can include documentation, meetings, mountains of mail to respond to, calls (some unpleasant) to return, appointments, management and staff pressures and conflicts, caseloads, workload, deadlines, and the relentless pressure of deadlines, all with no vacation time in sight. To be perfectly clear, burnout plays a very big role in compassion fatigue; however, its impact does not come close to that of compassion fatigue. Because of this, burnout alone has a better prognosis for recovery than compassion fatigue.

Compassion fatigue differs from burnout because compassion fatigue focuses on human suffering and tragedy on top of everyday work stress, which is the usual main component of burnout. Whereas burnout can result from any kind of repetitive or stressful work, compassion fatigue comes from treating and serving those who are suffering from the traumatic and crisis-driven events. With compassion fatigue, the caregiver experiences the emotional aftermath of a victimization or tragic loss, and these emotions or images often become difficult to discharge from the caregiver's thoughts. These images stay with the caregiver and very often invade the caregiver's life and thoughts.

BURNOUT AND COMPASSION FATIGUE: AN UNHOLY UNION

Beware when burnout and compassion fatigue happen together, because both conditions can exacerbate the other. For instance, witnessing or hearing about human suffering can overwhelm service providers so that they have great difficulty focusing and keeping up with the functional/administrative/documentation tasks their job requires. Sometimes this effect is often mistaken for procrastination. Conversely, a worker who faces conflicting and competing demands from management and/or systems and/ or the organizational loss of infra-structure and (changing) mission can experience a severe decline in purpose and morale, making it difficult for them to deal optimally with distressing client issues and scenarios.

In general, the average American worker labors under more stress than in years gone by. Stressors that include sales, competition, company growth, staff shortages, low wages, threat of job loss and threat of unemployment all impact the rank-and-file worker. Add to these the compounded stress caused by relationships, meeting family needs, fear of success or failure, traffic, road rage, and long lines waited in while buying services, food, supplies, and healthcare, is it any wonder that many workers suffer burnout and depression? And if anyone facing these stressors also works in the human services occupations, their risk of compassion fatigue grow exponentially.

NOW THAT YOU KNOW WHAT COMPASSION FATIGUE IS

Now that you know a little better what compassion fatigue is, and what it isn't, its relationship with PTSD and how it can exacerbate pre-existing conditions like burnout, you can be better able to spot compassion fatigue in yourself and others.

CHAPTER 4: CONTRIBUTING FACTORS TO COMPASSION FATIGUE

Your hand opens and closes, opens and closes. If it were always a fist or always stretched open, you would be paralyzed. Your deepest presence is in every small contracting and expanding, the two as beautifully balanced and coordinated as birds' wings. – Rumi, *The Essential Rumi*

This chapter will try to answer two questions, who is susceptible to compassion fatigue, and why. In other words, what are the contributing factors that can both cause and predispose someone to becoming a victim of compassion fatigue?

WHO IS SUSCEPTIBLE?

So first, who is susceptible to compassion fatigue? Generally, direct care service providers and family caregivers who deal with people who have experienced suffering and traumatic life experiences.

More specifically, here's an alphabetical list, by no means complete, of the kinds of direct care providers who are susceptible to compassion fatigue:

- Animal care service workers
- Caretakers for the elderly
- Child protective and welfare service workers
- Clergy
- Counselors
- Court-appointed specialist advocates
- Crisis response teams (i.e., rape crisis center workers)
- Emergency response teams, including fire and rescue, disaster workers and FEMA workers
- Family and youth service workers
- Family caregivers who care for spouses, elder parents, or loved ones
- Home health aids
- Hospice workers
- Judicial officers
- Medical and emergency staff, including nurses, doctors, and trauma unit staff
- Mental health service providers
- Parents (birth, foster, and kinship care) of children with serious physical, emotional, or mental illnesses and/or developmental challenges
- Police officers
- Probation staff
- Social workers
- Teachers and school based teams
- Therapists
- Veteran's counselors

THE MOST SUSCEPTIBLE: PEOPLE WHO WORK WITH CHILDREN

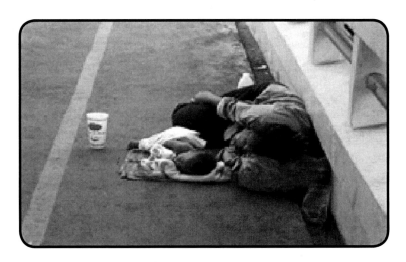

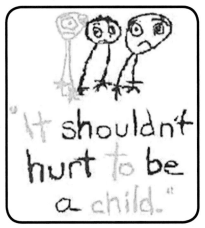

"It shouldn't hurt to be a child."

There is one population whose victimization or trauma seems to create more emotional distress than any other. As helpers, we are moved by adults of all ages who are vulnerable and in need of help. And when we witness or learn of the victimization of an adult or senior citizen, we feel deeply saddened for them and their families. But we are particularly distressed and even horrified by the traumatization of children, who are the most vulnerable in society. Traumatic events shouldn't happen to anyone, least of all children. The horror of child victimization can reverberate in our body and mind in the form of PTSD-like symptoms.

Child abuse and neglect is America's hidden epidemic. Of industrialized countries, the United States has the worst record of child abuse. Over 3 million reports of child maltreatment are made to state and local agencies each year—that's one report of abuse every 10 seconds (U.S. Department of Health and Human Services, 2010). Five children per day die as a result of this abuse (U.S. Department of Health and Human Services, 2011). Many children suffer a lifetime of abuse and while many children who suffer abuse are resilient, they live with the effects of abuse their entire lives. And the numbers continue to grow.

As these cases continue to increase, a number of factors including financial conditions impact the service systems that help our children who have become traumatized. Staff and resources have been drastically reduced at a time when they are needed more than ever. One result of shrinking resources during times of increasing demands for child welfare workers is higher caseload size which leads to emotional exhaustion of workers, increased staff turnover and lower service quality for children (Social Work Policy Institute, 2010). The average caseload for child welfare workers has been reported at between 24 and 31 children. All too frequently the numbers are often exceeding recommended levels, sometimes by double or more with a range in caseloads reaching as much as 100 children per worker while the Child Welfare League of America suggests a caseload ratio of 12 to 15 (Pearlman & Saakvitne, 1995).

Child protective services (CPS) and child welfare services are among the hardest impacted by secondary trauma. The professional groups most reflected include social workers, therapists, health care staff, psychologists, emergency response crisis teams, teachers, juvenile justice and judicial staff, court-appointed special advocates (CASA), probation staff, counselors, and clergy.

According to the National Child Traumatic Stress Network, the development of secondary traumatic stress (or compassion fatigue) is recognized as a common occupational hazard for professionals working with traumatized children. Studies show that from 6% to 26% of therapists working with traumatized populations, and up to 50% of child welfare workers, are at high risk of secondary traumatic stress or the related conditions of PTSD and vicarious trauma U.S. Department of Health and Human Services, Administration for Children and Families, Children's Bureau. (2011). Child Maltreatment 2010. Retrieved from http://www. acf.hhs.gov/programs/cb/stats_research/index.htm#can.

An important note: For those of you reading this book who have not worked in child welfare, I felt it important to state the following. Abuse in childhood has lifelong implications. Those of us working with troubled adults are often being challenged by the long-term consequences of child abuse manifesting in the adult sitting across from our desk, in a shelter, or behind bars. Deep in that adult is a child who did not receive the help they needed to escape their abuse, heal, and develop fully into the person they were meant to be.

In other words, when there is a shortage of dedicated child welfare workers (often due to un-managed compassion fatigue) there will be a tragic shortage of therapeutic interventions for these children, to their detriment and to the detriment of society.

And lastly, here are a few statistics to illustrate this concern. Up to 14% of male offenders and 37% of female offenders reported they had been physically or sexually abused before age 18. This is higher than the general U.S. population, where up to 8% of males and 17% of females were abused as children (Harlow, 1999). Some 59% of abused children are more likely to be arrested as a juvenile, while 28% are more likely to be arrested as an adult, and 30% are more likely to commit violent crime (Widom, Maxfield, 2001). And lastly, up to two-thirds of the people in treatment for drug abuse reported being abused or neglected as children (Fendrich, Mackesy-Amiti, Wislar, and Goldstein 1997). This does not have to be the case when we as a society help the remarkable people who are helping our children

IS EVERY CARE WORKER SUSCEPTIBLE?

Perhaps the lesson we can take away from this section is this: every direct care worker, from social worker to doctor to court-appointed therapist to firefighter is susceptible to compassion fatigue. Even if you don't happen to find your particular job title listed in this chapter but you work with those in crisis, you can be susceptible to compassion fatigue.

CONTRIBUTING FACTORS

Now that we know the large group of people who are susceptible to compassion fatigue, let's talk about some of the contributing factors that can lead to compassion fatigue.

LACK OF TRAINING

Nothing in our educational training or orientation can ever prepare us to handle every trauma our client's experience. For some of us, a culmination of client stories can rattle our ability to cope with job stress; for others, a single event can do the same.

Management must allot time during new staff orientations to educate about compassion fatigue. They can avoid significant staff confusion and distress when staff are taught to recognize compassion fatigue early on. Specialized training on compassion fatigue, self-regulatory skill development, crisis intervention, and the effects of trauma on children and adults can all help professionals anticipate challenges, understand their effects, and prepare professionals to deal with their clients' traumas.

HIGH IDEALS

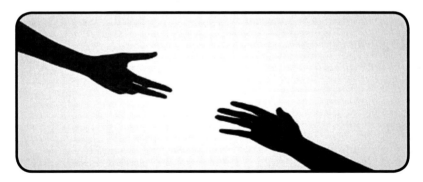

When I ask caregivers why they chose this field, many express a need to give back, to help, to make a difference, and to give others a chance for a better life. Next, when I ask them how often they get to see their best efforts help create sustained and lasting progress, all too often they answer, "not often enough." And then when I ask them how this leaves them feeling, they speak of frustration, self-doubt, disappointment, hopelessness, sorrow, exhaustion, and anger, even to questioning the point of it all.

As helping agents, we are wired to work hard on human issues and see clients progress to the next level, or come to some resolution. When this does not happen it exacerbates and/or creates significant stress in us.

EMPATHY AND COMPASSION

The love in our hearts can have great power. It can infuse us with a supernatural capacity to problem solve in our sleep, to rise from a poor night's sleep and tackle the new day, and to push past our depleted energies and keep working. It can also help us balance a phenomenal maze of chores, jobs, family members' needs, and social obligations.

Many, if not most, caregivers are empathetic and caring. Ironically, these necessary qualities that help us do our jobs also expose us to the pain, anger, and suffering of others, putting us in the direct path of experiencing Compassion Fatigue.

PEOPLE WHO ARE OVERLY DRIVEN BY LOVE

Sometimes love can be harmful. I'm not talking about fated romantic entanglements that go awry. Rather, I'm talking about the phenomenon of people who, driven by love, often care for others to the point of exhaustion. Driven by love, these people take on too much, forget to care for themselves, and forget to refill their own tank.

Sometimes I think in some peoples' hearts and lives, love can be addictive and can even act like adrenaline. Random House Webster's American Dictionary defines adrenaline as "a glandular secretion that speeds the heart; stirs one to action, etc." And if you're a caregiver who has felt that adrenaline rush, as it were, when you are driven by love to help, save and care for others, you may know what I'm talking about.

It is perhaps ironic that this same love, which drives us to help others, can turn on us when we see people in heartrending situations. There are times in our lives, both professionally and personally, when, driven by the love in our hearts, we persist in trying to fix a situation, regardless of how hard or hopeless it is, sometimes past the point of exhaustion. This attitude was what I was brought up with, and it was even written on my Father's headstone: "When things are not working, make it work!"

This same love can push rescue workers and law enforcement officers to move from one tragic, crisis-driven, and/or dangerous situation to another without stopping to count the personal cost. It can motivate clinical workers to work ceaselessly with a large volume of at-risk clients. It can move parents to hold all night vigils when a child is deeply troubled or suffering from an emotional or physical challenge, even when there will be no chance to rest the next day. And love can motivate family caregivers to manage multiple households and multiple lives to meet the demands of loved ones.

The point is, moved by love, we will try to improve the lives of those in need, even if it means overtaxing our own capacities. One could argue that as long as I have breath and am "doing," I have capacity. Yes, we do find the capacity to do what is needed. The bad news is, our body pays the price. There is a cost for caring for others when we neglect to also preserve our own wellbeing. Caring and empathy are qualities which are so needed in our world, but these same qualities can place us in the direct path for compassion fatigue. To avoid this trap we must love ourselves concurrent to the service that we have been called to do. We must honor that which is in us with self-care and be diligent in doing so.

"BUT I LOVE MY JOB!"

I sometimes hear this statement declared with a tinge of indignation when I am presenting on compassion fatigue or secondary and vicarious traumatization in the workplace. This declaration most often comes from someone new to child welfare. My challenge then is to explain to them how each of us who are called to this work have a strong sense of mission and passion, dedication, and purpose to do this work. However, the qualities of caring do not protect us from the risk factors embedded in the work.

The irony is that caring exposes us to risk, especially when we are unaware that diligent self-care must be a concurrent practice with caring for those in need. In my case, I love my work and I believed that because my work involved helping others that I would automatically be okay. The disconnect for me is realizing that the suffering and losses we are addressing touch us at the very core of our humanity; and this saddens, frustrates and frightens us. We are, however, often adept at dismissing the pain we feel focusing 100% on the pain in the persons we are helping. We are caring, helping people. Thus, we must learn early on to stay in touch with our humanity as well as our vulnerability to compassion fatigue.

All new job orientations should tell us that love, while vital to doing our jobs, will not protect us from the traumas we will experience. Instead, the same love that enables us to care for others also opens us to risk. When we finally realize this, we also realize that we must practice self-care habits to protect our wellbeing. By doing this we will also protect the love that we give.

YOUR OWN HISTORY OF TRAUMA OR VICTIMIZATION

Many helpers have personal histories or know someone close who has experienced trauma related to physical, emotional, sexual, or psychological victimization. When listening to a client telling of their (often similar) experience, this can cause the professional to experience a resurfacing of memories and emotions stored in both the mind and the body. The experience for the professional may be so intense that it activates many of the senses, thus recreating the sight, smell, touch, taste, and sound of their past victimization.

For example, as a child the author was chased and temporarily trapped by a stranger in an unsuccessful rape attempt. When listening to a client share a similar experience, I have at times experienced intense personal fear that was aligned with my past feelings of helplessness and entrapment. When that happens, I recognize the countertransference in myself and wrestle to put it in check so that I can stay present and helpful with my clients.

After recognizing our own issues, many caregiving professionals fall short of self-care and fail to talk with someone who can help us cope and heal. Instead, we re-experience these traumatic memories many times over as they are triggered by clients' stories. Many helping professionals try to bury disturbing personal content, which only allows it to resurface and reinjure us each time we hear a similar client story.

LACK OF CONSISTENT SELF-CARE HABITS

Many helpers fail to consistently practice self-care habits. As discussed earlier, these habits can help us manage and reduce the stress hormone that can flood into the brain and body several times a day. Many helpers also fail to periodically take the necessary time off of work, forgoing the health and rejuvenation that time off can provide.

In an attempt to manage our stress, many of us do try to go to the gym, take a walk, or engage in some fun activity, but we only do this once a week or even less. The problem with this is that after a week of intensely stressful work we often have stress hormone accumulated in our body. Waiting a whole week to engage in stress reducing activities to release these hormones is inadequate and unhealthy.

In another chapter we'll take a look at how the brain works and how the stress can travel and negatively impact your body if not managed adequately. The point I wish to drive home for you here is that because we have multiple stressors several times each day, we must therefore utilize techniques to reduce and manage that stress in our bodies several times a day, each day.

WORKING WITH LARGE NUMBERS OF TRAUMATIZED AND/OR VICTIMIZED PEOPLE

Let's look now at the intensity and frequency of stress events and how these impact stressors affect our minds and bodies. As mentioned earlier, the nature of the work we do often means that we experience traumatic stress almost daily. What happens to us when the intensity and frequency of the trauma we encounter becomes more than we can handle?

We are each unique in how traumatic stress impacts us. The physical and psychological symptoms we experience depend on personal variables, such as the level and consistency of care we give to our health and well-being, our capacity for dealing with multiple stressful events, prior experience, the degrees of exposure to certain types of stressors and the intensity, frequency, and nature of these events. How stress affects us can also be affected by our relationship to a victim and/or their family as well as our professional responsibility over their case.

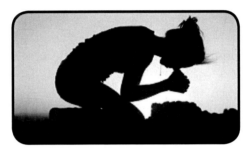

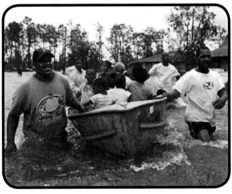

Some of our clients, in spite of our help, seem to be stepping off a cliff, while others are on the road to positive transformation. In an ideal world, each of us would have a caseload with a good balance of clients who are in crisis alongside those moving towards more positive outcomes, but that balance seldom exists.

Every story, event, and behavior of someone in crisis can cause us to have a traumatic stress response, and in our line of work, when we work with very frequent, high intensity crisis situations, which immerse us in traumatic content and experiences daily, we become vulnerable to being easily triggered. Being easily triggered, or in a state of hyper alertness in anticipation of the next crisis, changes us from calm people into people who now cannot be calm even in calm moments. Instead, we are constantly on edge, always expecting the other shoe to drop, always expecting another distressing experience.

Unlike with normal stressors, like waiting in a long checkout line or being stuck in traffic while late to get somewhere, where we can shake off the frustrations just experienced, the stressors in the intense work we do can cause sleepless nights, erratic mood swings, emotional shutdown, outbursts, anxiety, and depression, to name a few. Certainly, each individual employs unique coping mechanisms to navigate through others' pain and struggling. Just know that the coping mechanism you use changes you—how you perceive the world and operate in it.

THE CULTURES OF RELENTLESS SERVICE: OUR MESSAGES AND MODELS

Over many years of service I have had the honor and pleasure of working with a diverse group of people. They represent the Black cultures, Latin cultures, Native American cultures, Asian cultures, Middle Eastern cultures, and European cultures. When planning this book I thought that I might compare the level of self-care that each group in each culture engages in, contrasting those with propensity to engage in self-care against those who are relentless in their service and pay less attention to self-care. I realized that to do so would have been pretentious on my part as there are so many exceptions and variables within cultures, given the varying experiences and personalities of individuals within each culture. Our propensity to manage our self-care well, or not, doesn't seem to be linked to a particular culture.

More than the general culture where we grew up, our personalities and our coping styles also determine how we work through stressful situations. As children, we may not have been given permission to establish our own boundaries in terms of what works for us and what does not. The messages given us by family dynamics can even suppress our awareness that we have had enough and need to take a rest.

How we manage our self-care and who we become as helpers is shaped by many factors: the responsibilities placed on us early on, our communities and/or places of frequent fellowship, the people we live with, and other helpers that we closely observe. Many of these influences are very subtle, yet they can shape us. For example, within all cultures there are people with higher levels of tolerance for stress than others. Also, within all cultures people have unique perspectives, perceptions, and responses to the traumatized.

In my case, my father was always a kind and sensitive parent and was very concerned that we were able to be children and not push us into adult responsibilities prematurely, but one day he made a comment to me that, to this day, invites me to persist relentlessly in a problem when I should give it a rest. That day, my father, my sister and I were working hard trying to fix up a special space in our home for my mother who was returning from a brief hospitalization. I got tired and wanted to stop, so I plopped down on the couch and said "I'm tired. I'm done." My father, who had already worked his night shift by that time and had gotten my sister and I ready for school and dropped us off and then retrieved us from school, simply said to me "Don't be lazy—we have got to get everything ready for mommy."

He didn't accuse me of laziness; he simply admonished me not to be. However, I perceived it as letting him down. Over the years when I felt tired enough to stop I would hear his voice saying don't be lazy, and so I wouldn't stop. It was not just the words he said but the fact that I was looking at him knowing that he was exhausted too but he attended to the preparations for my mother with great detail, passion, and love. I felt ashamed of myself for simply wanting to stop helping. Throughout my adult life and still now on many levels I try hard not to let anyone down. I suspect many of you reading this share with me this driving force: a sometimes relentless determination to help.

Many of us also operate within the compounded responsibilities of caring for children *and* aging parents. This situation makes us even more vulnerable to compassion fatigue. It seems that those with the most complex and challenging and stressful responsibilities are the same people who invest enormous personal energy to help the less fortunate. This is because we get it; we relate so well to the struggles of others that we work relentlessly to ease their suffering and struggles. We just need to be careful that this compassionate work ethic doesn't lead to compassion fatigue.

PEOPLE, LIKE MYSELF, WHO HAVE TROUBLE SAYING NO

Many of the people I have talked to in my audiences agree that feelings of guilt often play a large role in their inability to say no. Some have told me that they feel ashamed of themselves when they don't respond to a need. And God forbid something more serious should happen to the needy had we only responded to their cry for help.

As I mentioned in the last section, my father's gently spoken admonishment not to be lazy implanted a powerful message that thereafter provoked feelings of guilt about letting people down. I am absolutely positive that was never his intent. I am also certain that for many of us the early imprinters in our lives did not intend for us to feel guilty when time out for self-care was needed. Not only did my father's words shape me, I was also shaped by the many people in my family and immediate circle I observed working tirelessly to help others. Often I could see they were tired and yet they pressed on with a smile, giving gentle words so that the people they were assisting would not feel badly about receiving their help.

And then there are those of us who simply need to be needed. Men and women alike have told me that they hate to feel useless. Many others have expressed a similar fear, which underlies their very purpose for existing. Some clergy have asked where are all of my people ? Some clergy are haunted by a fear of losing their congregation if they dare not to make every visit to the sick or respond to every phone request for help. Too often, clergy fail to delegate to ministry staff the task of meeting some of the one-on-one needs of their congregation.

THE ROLES GENDER MAY PLAY IN STRESS MANAGEMENT

Societal dictates that influence gender are at play here as well. Many women have been socialized to value the well-being of others over their own. When this happens, there can be no balance; rather, a one-sided focus of caregiving results. Men, on the other hand, generally do a better job of recognizing their limits. Men (perhaps with the exception of those in law enforcement and critical care) are more likely to sit down and refocus on something of interest to them, (e.g., some sport program or the paper) before resuming caring for others. This is not to say that they stopped caring. One caveat, however: while men may be more aware of their physical drain, too often they are not as sensitive to their emotional strains.

I illustrate this gender difference as a wake-up call to women. Too often when a woman is socialized to be self-neglectful, she risks becoming unaware of what she feels, which is detrimental to her physical and emotional health.

There are always exceptions to the rule. Within both genders are caregivers who possess stress-resistant personalities. These men and women tend to take much better care of themselves. We are the people that we are; however, whenever I run into people with healthy self-care habits I consistently try to take a page or two from their book. And I encourage you my readers who struggle in this area to do the same.

Discerning the distinction about this (need) is rather difficult when you consider your role as a counselor or a therapist, a social worker or part of the clergy, etc. and too few people come to you for help. Here we may be concerned that our services, our skills, our people connectivity serves limited or no benefit to others. And we can be misguidedly relieved when there is a constant flood of people lined up and waiting to see you. So how do you discern the difference between wanting to serve those in need, and needing to be needed? There's a fine line here but the latter places us in a vulnerable position to over extend ourselves to our detriment when we cannot say "enough for now" and take timeout to rest and recharge. In recent years, I have come to view some postponed events as a gift of time and I use them to recharge.

I often joke that those of us in the caregiving community seem to wear a big sign on our backs saying: "If you need anything, call me." This plays out when we finally get home after a challenging day at work and then answer the phone or receive unplanned visitation from friends, neighbors, or relatives who are requesting the last vestige of our energies to meet their needs. Many of us can't tell if those requests really demand our immediate attention or could possibly wait a bit and allow us some time to decompress from the battlefield we just stepped off of.

Many caregivers can't ignore more demands on our energies because we fear that we will lose people that matter to us if we request our own time to recover. While difficult and even painful for me, with the support and prompting of my accountability partners, I came to recognize that those who really care for me (and you) will respect my time and allow me a chance to rest and recover.

We must teach people how to treat us. When talking about this change with people with whom I had to make these changes, they told me that I had always given them the impression that I was readily available and able to help whenever they needed it. They never perceive me as tired and/or vulnerable. By me honestly sharing some of the challenges I faced in my work and my needs and plans for my time, they were able to appreciate that I needed downtime before taking on more issues. In fact, in a few rare cases, a couple of them assumed some role in monitoring more down time for me. Again, telling others that you need time away from caregiving is not easy to do. Sometimes I still have to catch myself, think more rationally, and take a self-inventory before saying yes, especially when I have been so conditioned from early on to say yes. However, it is crucial to learn to say no both in your personal and professional lives. I feel a great sense of relief when I postpone those things that can wait a while for me to take some "me time" to recharge my spirit, mind, and body.

SUMMING UP

As we can see, anyone in any of the direct service occupations can be susceptible to compassion fatigue, especially those who work with children in crisis. On top of that, each of us carries his or her own set of baggage that can make us more susceptible to compassion fatigue. In the next chapter, we'll talk about recognizing the symptoms of compassion fatigue, because recognizing the symptoms early leads to earlier intervention and treatment and can help minimize the effects of compassion fatigue.

CHAPTER 5:
RECOGNIZING THE SYMPTOMS

The awareness that health is dependent upon habits that we control makes us the first generation in history that to a large extent determines its own destiny.

–Jimmy Carter, *Everything to Gain*

If you're wondering whether you, or someone you know or care about, has compassion fatigue, this chapter will help you realize that there may be others, yourself included, who are either struggling with compassion fatigue or who are at high risk of developing it. I want to talk first about how compassion fatigue and stress manifest in our bodies. And then I will talk about how it affects our personal, professional, social, and spiritual lives.

HOW DOES COMPASSION FATIGUE MANIFEST IN OUR BODIES?

When the human body doesn't quickly integrate trauma, and the changes in the anatomy, biology, and neurology become chronic, the body becomes more vulnerable to trauma. The body loses its natural rhythms for regulating arousal and relaxation, entering a seesaw between hyper arousal and hypo arousal, which moves the person from explosive emotions to numbness, fatigue, detachment, and isolation.

When we have allowed too much stress to accumulate and exacerbate in our neurophysiology, our ability to tolerate even moderate or minor challenges and stressors decreases. We may find ourselves suddenly very angry or upset over something that is typically a minor issue, unable to understand why or how we've reached such an intense level of emotion.

When we lose our natural rhythm, we can swing from hyper to hypo (fight or flight) in a matter of minutes. This resembles rapidly changing mood swings and highs and lows in our energy. Picture also, when you find yourself needing to stay very busy, highly agitated, and needing to keep doing something. And then, in just a matter of moments, you feel completely washed out with no energy.

I was one of those people who could be completely shut down one moment and then all over the place busy the next moment. When I felt agitated, I would even create things to do, like rearranging my closets or my dishes, housecleaning, throwing things out, or shifting the furniture around in a room. It was very difficult for me to tell if I needed stimulation or rest. What I really needed was to step back, take stock of myself, and check in with someone to help me regulate myself.

STRESS HORMONE TRAJECTORY

The following paragraphs each describe a part of the brain involved with stress events and also chart the stress hormone trajectory that occurs when we experience stress. These descriptions can help us understand how stress affects our brain's and body's functioning so that we can better address, mitigate, and hopefully prevent the more damaging effects of compassion fatigue.

A QUICK CAVEAT

Please note that the following explanations are not intended to be exhaustive of all of the stress systems and responses. These systems have multiple functions and overlap in their roles with other areas in the brain and body. Please also note that the study of the brain is ever evolving, and my goal is merely to encourage and motivate you to engage in proactive self-care as you help others.

AMYGDALA

The Amygdala is made up of two almond-shaped concentrations of neurons located in our brain. It is important in the processing of memories and emotions. The amygdala is the first receiver and responder to every stressor and helps us stay safe and survive by warning the brain and the body of potential threats. During a stress event, it initiates the stress hormone which acts as a cellular communicator to alert the mind-body systems to take action for or avoid certain actions for our safety and survival. I like to compare it to a little guy in us who says "Oh Oh! Something is happening!" It may alert us not to walk down a particular alley or warn us that a car is rapidly approaching and we need to get out the way or let us know that a client interaction is escalating and that we should step back from or terminate it. The amygdala does not discern between positive stress signal events (such as "Surprise! It's your birthday!") and a real threat.

HIPPOCAMPUS

Also part of our brain, the hippocampus receives communications from the amygdala and distinguishes if the alert is a threat to our safety or a manageable situation. When it is clear that the situation or event is manageable and nonthreatening, the hippocampus modulates the amount of stress hormone flooding the brain and body. In other words, the hippocampus allows our brain chemistry under these conditions to return quickly to a state of calm.

When we stay in chronic and prolonged states of stress, however, the hippocampus is unable to modulate the stress hormone that is flooding it, and its capacity to function is greatly diminished. When this happens, the chemistry in our brains creates a state of dysregulation: we have reached levels of stress that is outside of our windows of tolerance.

The following are the four primary functions of the hippocampus:

1. Rational thought
2. Critical thinking
3. Problem-solving
4. Short-term memory

Given the importance of these key functions in our professional and personal lives, you need to make reducing and managing the amount of stress hormone that floods your systems a top priority.

ORBITOFRONTAL CORTEX

The orbitofrontal cortex (OFC), is the command center of the brain and governs the higher social, emotional, and behavioral functions as it receives communications from the hippocampus. When the hippocampus is functioning optimally, the communication to the OFC allows us to respond to threats and stress situations in a calm and mindful way.

But if the communication is coming from an overwhelmed or a diminished hippocampus (again due to persistent flooding of the stress hormone) feelings of fear and helplessness may result as the brain attempts to remain in a survival mode. The OFC drives our thinking to be reactive and can lead to avoidance behaviors such as isolation, negative thinking, withdrawal, flight, fight, and sleeplessness. It can also lead to hyperactivity, blaming, projection, anger, accident proneness, or impatience. When we are acutely or chronically overwhelmed with the stress hormone we do not do our best thinking. And instead of mindful responses to a situation, we often react in ways that we later regret. During the times when I failed to manage my daily stressors, I would often later say to myself—usually when I was lying awake in bed struggling to get to sleep—"I wish I could've handled that so much better." And I could have, if only my body and brain had not been flooded with stress hormones and I been able to think the situation through more clearly.

NEUROCIRCUITRY

At the same moment stress hormones communicate with brain systems, they also enter the body, traveling down the neural-circuitry into the stomach, creating what is commonly referred to as a "gut" reaction.

The stress hormone chemicals then proceed to various areas of our bodies where each person may uniquely experience the discomforts of stress. Examples of this may be butterflies or a tight full sensation in the abdominal area, stiffness and pain in the neck, tightness in the chest, throbbing or aching at the temples of our heads or behind our eyes, or tightness and clenching in the jaw, etc.

When stress hormones enter the body too often, significant and serious illnesses often results. So, when stress hits the body systems, the amygdala, as first responder, sends an alert for our survival. The body then automatically constricts until it gets a communication from the hippocampus that there is no real threat; that the situation is manageable. But when we allow multiple stressors to accumulate and exacerbate one upon another throughout the day and beyond, the constriction remains and possibly grows tighter. This constriction then (among other things) diminishes the healthy flow of healthy oxygen rich blood to all systems and organs. Therefore, it is imperative that we use relaxation techniques and strategies multiple times throughout the day to combat this constriction in our bodies. Later in this book I will illustrate in more detail the symptoms and health risks directly resulting from this condition.

THE NEUROSCIENCE OF TRAUMATIC STRESS

The above description of the neuro-physiological stress responses is deliberately basic and is not meant to be a comprehensive discussion of the highly complex brain stress activities. Part of what makes the modern field of neuroscience so fascinating is that research and understanding of the brain continually evolves. My aim is to provide all readers and listeners with a basic understanding of what may be happening and what we can do to self-regulate during the chronically and intensely stressful situations that are part of our service. So, for those of you who prefer a slightly more scientific explanation with more scientific terms, I have added the following:

According to neuroscientist Daniel Jay Goleman, who wrote the book *Emotional Intelligence* and is a psychologist and science journalist, the amygdala is responsible for registering and acknowledging any fear-based stimulus. Neuro transmissions then travel rapidly via a complex network to one or more sensory ports (e.g., the eyes or ears). The stress response is aroused before the cerebral cortex can even decipher the cause of the fear (Goleman, 1995).

According to Dr. Anna Baranowski and Teresa Lauer, LMHC, in their book *What is PTSD?: 3 Steps to Healing Trauma*, the hippocampus stores memories of perceived threats and their associated triggers. When we discern any trigger or threat, our mind and body prepares to respond. This process can go awry when we are continually responding to threats without any time in between each to calm or self-regulate. Traumatic memories are stored along with negative emotions (Baranowski & Lauer, 2012).

Trauma specialist Bryan Post states that when the hippocampus is continually flooded with the stress hormone (mostly cortisol), it cannot modulate the flow and thus cannot function to help us think critically and rationally, problem-solve, and access our short term memory (Post, 2002). Dr. Baranowski explains it this way: "After exposure to a disturbing event, the body and mind send signals that activate the adrenal glands which pump out high levels of the stress hormone, cortisol. Too much cortisol short-circuits the cells in the hippocampus, making it is harder to organize the memory of the trauma or the stressful experience" (Baranowski & Lauer, 2012).

Dr. Goleman also states that, "When stimulus perceived as a threat is picked up by the cerebral cortex, an alarm goes off and the body goes into survival mode which is a state of physical constriction and emotional discomfort. It is beneficial to employ techniques wherein we are able to temporarily deactivate the senses long enough for our bodies to achieve a state of homeostasis and calm" (Goleman, 1995).

The two senses most frequently activated by stress are hearing and sight. Thus, the tools most often useful for calming involve visual imagery and music.

Most importantly, by intentionally and consistently employing self-care strategies (which may include professional or friendly help from others) and techniques, we can create the changes in our brain chemistry necessary to regulate ourselves.

LIST OF POSSIBLE SYMPTOMS AND SIGNS IN YOUR PROFESSIONAL LIFE

Now let's move out of our brain and body and see how stress and compassion fatigue affect our daily lives. The following is a (non-exhaustive) list of compassion fatigue signs and symptoms as they manifest at work and in our professions. The more you know about these symptoms, the better you can spot compassion fatigue, even in its beginning stages, in yourself and your coworkers. In most cases, the person who is starting to suffer from compassion fatigue is often the last person to recognize it.

Additionally, when you recognize these signs in others, you will know that these uncharacteristic and at times negative behaviors are caused by the compassion fatigue, rather than by any character defect in the sufferer. I challenge you to become a "loving meddler" by being aware of the emotional and behavioral changes in other direct care workers around you. Knowing that those changes are most often stress related, rather than a sign of an intentionally and unnecessarily difficult person, you will be better able to step in and offer your support, counsel, and assistance.

- Low morale
- Task avoidance
- Obsession with details
- Apathy
- Decreased motivation
- Negativity
- Diminished appreciation in formerly joyful activities
- Detachment
- Poor work commitment
- Staff conflict
- Absenteeism
- Irritability
- Withdrawal from colleagues
- Loss of confidence

MORE DETAIL: HOW THESE SYMPTOMS PRESENT IN OUR PROFESSIONAL LIVES

The following is a detailed description of each of the listed symptoms as they manifest at work, along with an explanation of how they are often mistakenly viewed by those who are not aware of compassion fatigue. One thing to note: as you read the following symptom descriptions, you may notice that many of them seem to overlap. This is testimony to the dynamic nature of compassion fatigue itself. Its symptoms are many and its effects are wide-ranging.

Low morale: This may stem from diminished sense of purpose, sense of mission, enthusiasm and energy to do the work. What others may see is a marked withdrawal from team participation and other work related activities, which can be mistaken for laziness or irresponsibility.

Task avoidance: This can occur naturally when the task is associated with a prior traumatic experience. The worker who may be shielding herself from further distress needs some time to be able to process and manage the distressful event. This behavior may be mistaken for the irresponsibility, pawning off work onto others, or laziness.

Obsession with details: The worker may be fearfully focusing on work details that they perceive to hold the whole together, being unable to see the bigger picture in disturbing situations. This behavior can annoy coworkers who may experience this behavior as micromanagement, procrastination, or needless attempts at perfectionism.

Decreased motivation: When your enthusiasm has turned sour, you experience your clients as irritants instead of persons. You may feel very negative about work, complain frequently, avoid tasks, avoid talking about what you do, or see your work efforts as futile. Sometimes this has mistakenly been perceived as unfitness for the job.

Apathy: The worker appears not to be affected by a traumatic event. A worker can become (or appear) apathetic as a way to protect themselves from further injury from the trauma suffered by their clients. This is potentially problematic as the worker is not exercising two key elements necessary to heal: (1) Integrating the traumatic situation, and (2) processing the experience's impact on themselves. In fact, by blocking further injury they end up locking initial secondary traumatic material inside. In this case, I urge their coworkers to become involved (meddle!) and encourage the suffering worker to open up and release what is going on.

Negativity: The negative worker's hopelessness can turn into anger and possibly rage. For them, the world becomes increasingly perceived, experienced, and viewed in dark terms. They may even harbor feelings of disgust for people in general. They may begin to view those around them who are struggling as ignorant or incompetent or intentionally sabotaging their own progress. Patience is lost. Humor is absent, and having fun is not even on the radar. Often, coworkers will avoid a negative worker. However, a worker in this state needs kind yet persistent help to nudge them forward, someone to shine a positive light on work situations and life in general.

Diminished appreciation in formerly joyful activities: The worker loses interest in activities that formerly gave them pleasure: e.g., the arts, outdoors, reading, hobbies, music, visiting friends and family, social activities, anything fun. They find it difficult to see good or beauty in any situation. Others may experience the worker as one who says no to every fun idea, and who is thankless, sullen, angry and unapproachable. When I was suffering from compassion fatigue, I am told that I was not sullen, angry, or unapproachable. Rather, I appeared to be focused only on work and nothing else. For myself, I needed to be pulled back into activities that I formerly enjoyed. For instance, my son bought me paint brushes and canvasses and declared: "Mommy, it's time." Out of appreciation of his insight and kindness, and the very generous amount of money he spent, I took a shot at some painting and then became hooked, creating several finished pieces. Other friends and loved ones pulled me into activities like theater, sightseeing, etc.

Detachment: The worker avoids others and disconnects from all aspects of work that remind them of painful experiences. This can include decreased communication, self-imposed isolation, increased absenteeism, tiredness, and poor concentration. This behavior is often mistaken for having a bad attitude, being uncooperative, or just not being a team player.

Poor work commitment: This is a loss of mission and purpose, often causing us to ask "why?" and "what is it all for?" Often this can stem from being chronically overwhelmed. These behaviors can be mistaken for poor work performance, poor follow through, and procrastination.

Staff conflict: This is common as workers begin to mistrust other team members. Self-doubt can cause them to perceive that their efforts are being sabotaged by clients, and/or coworkers or that they are being viewed negatively or as incompetent by management and coworkers. Tensions rise as workers desperately try to makes sense of situations that seem unresolvable, and blame and projection can often occur. This behavior is often mistaken as the worker acting difficult on purpose. Fear is a big part of the cause in workers who don't know what's happening to them or don't realize the impact secondary traumatic stress is having on them.

Absenteeism: This can occur as emotional and physical symptoms overtax and drain the worker's mind and body. The stresses that brought the worker to this point can incapacitate their bodies to the point of illnesses, robbing their strength, and making it difficult to face another day at work. Fatigue and exhaustion have taken their toll. According to Dr. Bruce Perry, unchecked compassion fatigue causes the body to wear down and ultimately wear out.

Exhaustion: This is fatigue beyond which is normal for the human body and mind. Like other symptoms, this may be mistaken for laziness, all to the detriment of the worker. If the worker remains exhausted for too long, they can become emotionally and physically depressed, which can lead to serious illness.

Irritability: Here, the worker becomes impatient and may cut corners to finish or avoid tasks and people they can no longer tolerate. In this state, the worker becomes short-tempered easily provoked to anger, demonstrating knee-jerk reactions to perceived insults or communications that challenge their ideas. Performance may decline due to frequent oversights, mistakes, and lapses in concentration. The worker may begin to mock clients and coworkers. They may also blame clients and even use inappropriate humor. This too is often viewed as unfitness for the job.

Withdrawal from colleagues: All too often, secondarily traumatized people isolate themselves and avoid contact with others. This is often caused by a fear of being viewed as less than capable if we share our problems with our peers. Sadly, this can leave us with no peer communication and no social life inside or outside of work. If we only realized that our problems are caused by stress, and not personal shortcomings, we might be more willing to share. Withdrawal can be mistaken for unfriendliness, arrogance, and an unwillingness to join the work team.

Loss of confidence: When working with troubled human beings, the nature of the work has many setbacks, disappointments, system constraints, limited resources, and sometimes failures. All of these can leave workers questioning their abilities. Compassion fatigue can keep the afflicted worker stuck in chronic self-doubt.

HOW COMPASSION FATIGUE AFFECTS OUR PERSONAL LIVES: COGNITIVE SYMPTOMS

The following is another non-exhaustive list of compassion fatigue symptoms, but this time it is of those that impact our mental functioning. Most symptoms are quite self-explanatory, so I will explain only those that seem to demand more explanation.

- Confusion
- Spaciness
- Trauma Imagery
- Rigidity
- Self-doubt
- Minimization
- Thoughts of harming self or others
- Disorientation

Trauma imagery: is the experience of a picture/flashback or a vision of a traumatic event that occurred on one of your cases; an assault or victimization in progress, or the aftermath of an act of violence. Consider the first ones on the scene immediately after the horrific shooting massacre in Aurora Colorado. The images of the carnage; severely and fatally wounded men women and children will replay in their minds many times over the years to come. Sometimes these images may come even when just reading a case history. I have spoken to many court personnel and various clinicians who have reported having a vision of someone's victimization/violation actually in operation before even seeing the victim. These images come just by reading the reports. The disturbing images may invade you repeatedly at any time or anywhere.

Rigidity: in thinking is where you may get stuck when you employ the same responses/interventions to a common occurrence in your work even though your actions have not previously been effective in generating positive outcomes and progress for the case. When under too much stress it can become very difficult to see the bigger picture or see things in more general themes. The pattern becomes so rigid that even after a colleague attempts to intervene and suggest some alternatives, it may be impossible for you to change your course of action. If we remember, when the hippocampus is flooded with stress hormone, critical thinking and problem solving is quite difficult to access.

HOW COMPASSION FATIGUE AFFECTS OUR PERSONAL LIVES: EMOTIONAL SYMPTOMS

Emotional symptoms of compassion fatigue can be some of the most damaging. An acquaintance of mine who worked many years in a juvenile hall found a youth who hanged himself in his cell. My acquaintance was further horrified after realizing that the other juvenile inmates simply sat by and watched the hanging without calling for help. This acquaintance handled/managed the whole situation efficiently, and appeared to be coping with the tragedy. However, he did not discuss or process it; instead, he stuffed the incident deep inside and went about his work. Over the next few months, he unwittingly created a climate of discord both at work and at home that ultimately damaged his work and home life relationships with his co-workers, his spouse, and especially his children.

Had he talked about this horrific event, and had he been encouraged by others to process the experience and its impact on himself, key areas of his personal and professional life might have remained intact.

Here then, is a list of emotional symptoms of compassion fatigue to watch out for:

- Anxiety
- Emotional roller coaster
- Anger
- Rage
- Numbness
- Overwhelmed
- Fear
- Depression
- Depleted energies
- Sadness
- Survivor's guilt

As before, some of the symptoms need no further explanation. I have expanded on a few that might require more explanation.

Emotional roller coaster: This shows up as an inability to regulate one's own states of arousal leading to a rapid seesawing between numbness to explosive emotional states. We recognize these states as being hyper or hypo or fight or flight. In general, we witness these states in children when we see the boys being too hyper (active) and the young girls being more hypo (e.g., withdrawn and quiet). We also generally witness this in adults when we women get very busy cleaning and rearranging things to calm ourselves. Conversely we can see this in men when they settle down to watch a game or read a newspaper, which can be a form of retreating.

Where we differ in heightened states of traumatic stress, is that we rapidly swing from one state to the other sometimes in a matter of minutes, finding it very difficult to regain or maintain a state of calm.

Depression: This is seen most often in the cases of committed workers in the human services. This is best described as a functional depression wherein we can perform all responsibilities close to or at our normal energy level. However, we do so while carrying an undercurrent of sorrow and negative feelings, thus creating an internal heaviness that drains our energy resources in an unhealthy way. In this state, our bodies are being dragged along by our sheer determination without the physical reserves necessary for our wellbeing.

Depleted energies: As caregivers, we not only expend much mental and physical energy, we also tend to stay on high alert throughout the day and beyond because it is difficult to wind down and decompress. We then carry work concerns when we should be resting and restoring ourselves, often without being aware that we are doing so. As a result, we deplete our internal resources and compromise our ability to cope effectively with the continued demands of serving those deeply in need.

HOW COMPASSION FATIGUE AFFECTS OUR PERSONAL LIVES: BEHAVIORAL SYMPTOMS

Here's a quick list of how compassion fatigue affects us and manifests itself in our behaviors. Again, most of these are pretty self-explanatory, but I have added detail for a few that needed further explanation.

- Clingy
- Moody
- Nightmares
- Impatient
- Appetite changes

- Hyper vigilance
- Elevated startle response
- Use of negative coping
- Sleep disturbance

Appetite changes: for many, stress creates a loss of appetite. For many more, consuming more food and drink is a way to cope with stress. Significant amounts of stress hormone deplete the body of much needed nutrients thereby creating cravings of certain foods (salty, sugary, refined carbs) or sugary and tart/alcoholic beverages.

Hyper vigilance: This is a state of continuous anticipation, scanning the environment for the next crisis. People experiencing this often say things like "what else can go wrong?" or "it's quiet now, but this won't last." Being in this ramped up state of mind activates the amygdala and sends more of the stress hormones into the brain and body.

Elevated Startle Response: You are at home and you know that your family is in the house. Yet, when someone suddenly walks into a room where you are preoccupied, you jump out of your skin. You are in a heightened survival mode and have just experienced a perceived threat to safety, even though you are safe. This is common with compassion fatigue.

Sleep disturbances: If you wake up in the morning tired and perspiring, with your bed disheveled beyond the normal and your sleepwear twisted around you, you may be experiencing sleep disturbances. In other words, you are mentally wrestling with unfinished business or traumatic events during your sleep. In this state, you are not experiencing adequate Rapid Eye Movement, REM sleep; the sleep level where our bodies get to rest and rejuvenate. This can lead to sleep deprivation, which, if chronic, can compromise your health and safety, especially while driving.

HOW COMPASSION FATIGUE AFFECTS OUR PERSONAL LIVES: SPIRITUAL LIVES

Here's a quick list of how compassion fatigue affects our spiritual lives. Again, most of these are pretty self-explanatory, so instead of explaining each, I am including a story of a woman who dealt with her spiritual challenges.

- Loss of purpose
- Anger at God
- Questioning prior religious beliefs
- Pervasive hopelessness

SPIRITUALITY IS UNIVERSAL

Many of us at some time in our lives have had experiences which can best be described as spiritual. And each of us has a set of beliefs about the world and humanity and our own way to express this core part of ourselves. Included here is a brief picture from a very special children's services worker named Mary, and later, my own spiritual Journey in caregiving service to humanity.

Spirituality: The very essence or anchor for many of our lives and the part that informs us that we are not alone: we are loved, supported, protected, cared for, made whole, and one with all creation. This is the part of us we should feed, nurture, and refresh with all diligence. And when it has been nurtured and fed, it is the part of us best equipped to replenish, recharge, and restore us to peace, joy, and inner calm.

When our spirituality is impacted by compassion fatigue, we can lack the ability to re-connect with our purpose, be strong in our faith, access our source, and draw on the strength necessary to meet daily challenges.

MARY'S STORY

Mary attended one of my workshops, and at the end she hugged me and wept bitterly about the pain and frustration she felt about her experiences in the child welfare field. First, she stated that so much of what I said in a workshop connected with her powerfully and that she had struggled with many of the symptoms I described and would now try to practice the strategies I taught to help herself. However, she felt helped only to the extent that she now knew better how to take care of herself.

Mary's anguish lay in her struggles with the work itself. She served children five years old and younger who had been brutally sexually assaulted. She was horrified about the numbers of these cases as they poured in.

Mary was also very distressed about the apparent lack of help available for these babies (as she called them) and it seemed to her that nobody cared enough to help the children. She especially questioned what she was doing: was she making any difference at all?

Helping children who are sexually brutalized is one of the most difficult areas to work in. It is beyond comprehension why precious and vulnerable innocence is destroyed at the hands of people, many of them their parents and caregivers. We can never do enough to protect our children, and so it is natural to feel uncertain that we are really doing anything to help them in the aftermath of such devastating violations and injuries that can happen. Coming face to face with this level of evil and cruelty would cause many of us to question our faith, beliefs, and understanding of humanity.

I asked Mary what she does when she sees a child so brutally injured in this way, and she says in addition to her professional tasks, she holds them and hugs them when she is able. I said to her then that is what you get to do: to hold them close to your heart so that those injured souls can feel and hear the beat of your heart and feel the safety of your arms and love emanating from your spirit. I asked her to try not to expend her energy agonizing or being angry over system-wide issues outside of her control. I encouraged her to realize that she gets to give those precious children a few moments embraced in her love. I asked Mary to realize that in addition to her duties, she is a brief but essential healing balm for traumatized children. I next strongly encouraged her to seek ongoing professional counseling to help her process the stresses of her work, for her own sake as well as to remain available to these children who need her love and clinical skills.

HOW COMPASSION FATIGUE AFFECTS OUR PERSONAL LIVES: INTERPERSONAL SYMPTOMS

Here's a quick list of how compassion fatigue affects us and manifests itself in our interpersonal relationships. Again, most of these are pretty self-explanatory, but I have added detail for a few that needed further explanation.

- Withdrawal
- Overprotective
- Mistrust

- Decrease in Sexual Intimacy
- Isolation
- Projection of anger and blame
- Intolerance
- Loneliness

Some of the experiences you may have are interpersonal and involve relationships with others.

Decrease in Sexual Intimacy: chronic and prolonged stress can deplete our energies to the extent that our most basic biological force, the libido, becomes suppressed. Our libido is a powerful force of life energy that sparks our zeal, creativity, passions, and excitement to connect with and enjoy all that life has to offer. Sexual energy and desire is part of the libido. When diminished much or most of the flame may go out.

Loneliness: The overwhelmed state of stress often places us in an emotional space where we feel alone in our struggles with the demands placed on us. This is compounded by a tendency to refuse to ask for help because we assume that no one could possibly understand how we feel. We can feel completely alone even while surrounded by many people. Often, loneliness can be self-imposed, as was my case because I did not reach out to people when I needed to actively be in their presence and fully engaged.

Intolerance: This is an inability to tolerate even minor annoyances that, under calmer states, we would be able to manage. Traumatic stress makes it difficult to regulate our states of arousal (fight or flight), causing us to go numb or become combative or explosive with little or no provocation when confronted with everyday stresses.

HOW COMPASSION FATIGUE AFFECTS OUR PERSONAL LIVES: PHYSICAL SYMPTOMS

Some of the personal experiences you may have involve our physical health. Here then is a quick list of how compassion fatigue affects us and manifests itself in our physical wellbeing. Again, most of these are pretty self-explanatory, but I have added detail for a few that needed further explanation.

- Aches
- Pains
- Shock
- Dizziness
- Breathing difficulties
- Somatic Complaints
- Impaired immune system
- Rapid heartbeat

Somatic complaints: These are bodily discomforts that can include aches, pains, burning or tingling sensations, itches, tightness, and many more. Given the importance early intervention, it's good to realize that these are warning signs that we need to take care of our bodies.

Impaired immune system: This is considered by many to be the most at risk system in the body as a result of unmanaged traumatic stress. Because this system can become impaired and even shut down by traumatic stress, it makes our bodies highly susceptible to many illnesses with limited or no ability to fight off viruses and infections, for example: the flu, pneumonia, an open wound, inflammation, or the common cold.

As stated earlier, the above is not an exhaustive list, yet it points to some of the more prevalent symptom impacts of compassion fatigue. Though stated as symptoms, I urge you to look upon these as indicators: early warning signs you need to address as soon as possible to avert damage to you and your coworkers' emotional and physical health. Early intervention is the hallmark of wellness for those who help others.

PROFESSIONAL QUALITY OF LIFE SURVEY, OR PROQOL

The Professional Quality of Life Survey, or ProQOL, is a wonderful tool available to help you evaluate yourself for compassion fatigue. Beth Hudnall Stamm, Ph.D., developed the ProQOL questionnaire that measures your levels of compassion satisfaction, compassion fatigue (or secondary traumatic stress) and burnout. It is statistically reliable and has been shown to help professionals. I highly recommend that you take the questionnaire, which I have included below. After you take the questionnaire, please read my explanations on how to score it. Please note: when the question asks about you and those you work with, it's not referring to co-workers, but rather to your clients (i.e., suspects, offenders, victims, patients, etc.) and related family members that you interview and supervise.

Please use a separate piece of paper and a pencil and write each question number along with your numerical response (i.e., #1-4 #2-5, etc.).

PROFESSIONAL QUALITY OF LIFE SCALE (PROQOL) COMPASSION SATISFACTION AND COMPASSION FATIGUE, VERSION 5 (2009)

When you help people you have direct contact with their lives. As you may have found, your compassion for those you work with can affect you in positive and negative ways. Below are some questions about your experiences, both positive and negative, as a service provider. Consider each of the following questions about you and your current work situation. Select the number that honestly reflects how frequently you experienced these things in the last 30 days.

ProQOL 1-10

1 =Never 2=Rarely 3=Sometimes 4=Often 5=Very Often

1. I am happy.
2. I am preoccupied with more than one person I work with.
3. I get satisfaction from being able to help people.
4. I feel connected to others.
5. I jump or am startled by unexpected sounds.
6. I feel invigorated after working with those I help.
7. I find it difficult to separate my personal life from my life as a service provider.
8. I am not as productive at work because I am losing sleep over traumatic experiences.
9. I think that I might have been affected by the traumatic stress of those I work with.
10. I feel trapped by my job as a service provider.

ProQOL 11-20

1 =Never 2=Rarely 3=Sometimes 4=Often 5=Very Often
11. Because of my work, I have felt "on edge" about various things.
12. I like my work as a helping professional.
13. I feel depressed because of the traumatic experiences of the people I work with.

14. I feel as though I am experiencing the trauma of someone I have worked with.
15. I have beliefs that sustain me.
16. I am pleased with how I am able to keep up with helping techniques and protocols.
17. I am the person I always wanted to be.
18. My work makes me feel satisfied.
19. I feel worn out because of my work as a

    _____.

20. I have happy thoughts and feelings about those I help and how I could help them.

ProQOL 21-30

1 = Never 2= Rarely 3= Sometimes 4= Often 5= Very Often
21. I feel overwhelmed because my case work load seems endless.
22. I believe I can make a difference through my work.
23. I avoid certain activities or situations because they remind me of frightening experiences of the people I work with.
24. I am proud of what I can do to help.
25. As a result of my work in the helping professions, I have intrusive, frightening thoughts.
26. I feel "bogged down" by the system.
27. I have thoughts that I am a "success" as a professional_____
28. I can't recall important parts of my work with trauma victims.
29. I am a very caring person.
30. I am happy that I chose to do this work.

SCORING THE PROQOL: COMPASSION SATISFACTION

When scoring this section, you'll be looking at the numerical answers you entered for each of the questions in this scale and then finding the total. There highest score you can get on this scale is 50 (answering each of the 10 questions with a 5) and the lowest score you can obtain is a 10 (answering all 10 questions with a 1). If your score was 22 or less, you are in the low range of compassion satisfaction, suggesting that you are not deriving pleasure or joy from your work. If your score was between 23 and 41, your level of compassion satisfaction is in the average range when compared to others in helping professions. If your score is 42 or more, you seem to be experiencing a high level of job satisfaction and feel confident and positive about the contribution you're making to your profession.

SCORING THE PROQOL: BURNOUT

This section is scored a little differently. Once you check each of your answers to the questions listed below, the ones in red will reverse in order to calculate an accurate score. So if you answered question #1 with a 5, you would change that 5 to a 1, and if you answered it with a 2, you would change that score to a 4, and so on.

Scoring 22 or less on this scale indicates that you are operating at a low level of burnout. This suggests that you are comfortable in your work environment and feel engaged, in control, and able to handle the demands of your job. If you scored from 23 to 41, you are in the average range of burnout when compared to others in helping professions. If you scored 42 or higher, it appears that you are in the high range of burnout, indicating that you are probably feeling detached, overwhelmed, or hopeless about your work contribution and your work environment.

SCORING PROQOL: SECONDARY TRAUMA SCALE

No reversals are required in the scoring of this section. Just score each of your answers to the following questions as they appear on your answer sheet and then add them up. Again, the highest score would be a 50, and the lowest would be a 10.

A score of 22 or less on this secondary trauma scale indicates that your level of stress is low. You're probably able to objectively work with the traumatic issues that come up at work and are able to balance your personal life with your life at work. If you scored between 23 and 41, you are working at an average rate of secondary trauma when compared to others in helping professions. A score of 42 or higher indicates that you are at a high rate of secondary trauma and may be feeling fragile, frightened, or consumed with negative thoughts and images related to the trauma of those you work with.

WHAT DO THESE SCORES MEAN TO YOU?

It's important to remember that this survey was a quick look at how you're feeling right now about yourself and your work. It is not a diagnostic tool and is not meant to imply that problems exist whenever someone has an elevated score. The instrument is reliable and has been validated, and the studies were normed on cross section of helping professionals. It is important to note that in the cases of law enforcement, scoring may average a little differently than other helping professionals. In addition, for all helping professionals, you may be dealing with a specific issue that can affect your score today, and the instrument does not take those personal issues into consideration.

So having cautioned you about the scores, I still suggest that you consider your scores, think about any discomfort you feel at work that's associated with either burnout or secondary traumatic stress, and then pay close attention to the many strategies and suggestions I'll be offering about how to lower stress levels that result from compassion fatigue. Of course, I also encourage you to seek professional assistance if you find yourself having difficulty processing the information from this manual on your own.

RECOGNIZING THE SYMPTOMS, A LIFELONG COMMITMENT

As you can see, there are many many symptoms and ways that compassion fatigue manifests itself in our professional and personal (cognitive, emotional, behavioral, spiritual, interpersonal, and physical) lives. Now that you are becoming aware of these symptoms and know better what to watch out for, I hope you are realizing that as a caregiver you have a lifelong commitment to monitor your health as well as support the health of those you work with.

CHAPTER 6:
STORIES FROM THE FIELD

Trying to please everyone else, you are never in your life going to be happy. If people learn to stand up and say NO, they will be a lot happier. You can't please everyone. If you set out to please everybody, you are going to be the one who is miserable.

–Madea [Tyler Perry],
Madea's Unlimited Comments on Love and Life

Sometimes, the best way to understand a phenomenon like compassion fatigue is to hear others' stories about it, especially when those stories come from other direct care workers. Each of these stories in this chapter is from an experienced worker who has labored under some of the stressors we've discussed. Their stories might help you realize that compassion fatigue is something all direct care workers have to deal with. Also, each story is an example of the volatile combination of burnout and secondary distress that impact many dedicated caregivers.

BETTY'S STORY

Betty is an LCSW and Master Life Coach. As a social worker with 25 plus years of experience, the challenges she has faced are complex. The missions and the systems she worked in were in stark competition. Betty wisely examined all areas of her life and, using personal insight, made a decision to care for her own well-being.

My specialty is life transitions and assisting those in need (which is what I also do as a life coach). I have worked in shelters both runaway and transitional for children and homelessness. I am a medical social worker and have worked ER, Infectious Disease, Hospice and Home Health: I have worked extensively with foster children and started the current Alameda County Wraparound program Project Permanence for Lincoln Child Center; I conduct clinical supervision at Easy Bay Alameda County and have had a private practice as well.

I was born to be a healer and as a child I thought I would be a doctor, but college showed me that it was not the physical, but the social, emotional, and spiritual piece which needed to be addressed most. I have always worked with children and have also worked with illness, death, and dying. I feel that life transitions are the most challenging for us as we are not always in alignment with the changes these transitions require. The pivotal point for me was when I lost a friend to an aneurism: more than the debilitating condition, I was devastated by an unjust and prejudicial system that prevented my friend from getting the medical care she needed, which themselves became factors that resulted in her death. I feel that our social services structure is fragmented and challenging to negotiate for those in need. I firmly believe I am a change agent, meant to heal on all levels. To that end, I also became an ordained minister as well to fully embrace the needs of all people to the best of my ability.

One of my most distressing experiences occurred when I was a medical social worker. For part of my job, I worked as the infectious disease social worker for a children's hospital in a neighboring state. The job also entailed working at that county's level 5 trauma center helping the HIV positive parents of the same children I already worked with at the children's hospital. On top of that, I also worked at a clinic that cared for HIV positive teens in my own state. This was my dream job, one which I had wanted for years. It was also an opportunity to work with HIV positive children and families while providing care as a medical social worker. As a side note, the children's hospital was connected with the local university and conducted research on anti-retrial viral medications.

As a patient-centered social worker, your first concern should be your patients' physical and mental well being. At least, that's the ideal. But sometimes, the administration you work for has other priorities. In this case, I felt that the administration I worked for was only paying lip service to my clients' health and welfare, that their real priority was the research. The research division head actually did not want any changes to the way things had been running and wanted the program to remain with a strictly medical model of treatment where the child is treated as a number rather than an individual. I also was running into a problem with getting the needed time off. The department head of infectious disease did not think that I needed to use my accrued time because I was working with multiple departments as needed by the social work department. On top of this, a child life worker's had relocated to our team. This child life worker' mission was to help children affected by a ravaging disease and provide them home and quality care.

On the positive side, my work at the teen clinic and with the nurse managers located at the county hospital was fluid, rewarding. The coordination was seamless with the main nurse practitioner in charge.

Working with the children's clinic, however, was a different story. There, the head RN had long wanted to relocate to another department, having worked there for 10+ years, but the research and department head had blocked her transfer, which made her quite unhappy. For two years we provided the best service we could to our patients, supported the parents of infected children who were themselves also infected, and addressed their stabilization and daily choices, which affected their lives.

During this time, I began to experience sleep disturbances, hives, muscle tensions, and fatigue, all of them stress-related. I had a particular patient who was receiving treatment for lymphoma in conjunction with her anti retrial viral medications which were wreaking havoc on her system at the age of 16 years old as she had full blown AIDS by age 10.

I had another client, a mother, who was in jeopardy of losing her housing and her two children should she miss her Section 8 appointment. However, her viral load was so high it was creating HIV dementia in her system. She needed the evaluation and intake necessary to qualify for the anti-retroviral medications she had resisted taking. This mother was mentally unable to follow through and needed help making, showing up for, and following through with her appointments.

I helped this mother attend her Section 8 meeting and with her intake, and she was able to receive the necessary medications and think more clearly. My other client, the mother of the 16-year-old, needed help as well. After her child was clear of the lymphoma, I was informed that the child wanted to take a medication holiday lasting between a few weeks to less than three months to give her body a rest from the massive amounts of medications she had been given. This vacation would allow her body to rest and help her to eat and absorb good foods. As the medical social worker, I listened to her needs and conducted a psychosocial and mental status exam of the 16 year old patient. After this evaluation, I deemed her mentally competent to make such a decision with the support of her mother.

Sadly, my decision to allow her to take a medicine vacation did not fare well with the head research doctor. He pressured me to change my decision and pressured the medical staff to force the patient to continue her medication. He held an interdisciplinary team meeting, and within two weeks they overrode my decision, gave me a scathing review, and changed my job description in order to move me out of the children's clinic.

At this time, I was seeking medical attention using eastern methods as my body would not respond to western treatments. I walked regularly and studied kickboxing for exercise. But it was too much and too late. After a bottle of Ouzo (a Greek alcoholic beverage) and a few mental health days off, I decided to look after my health needs first and find work easier on my health and more in line with my belief system.

Had I to do this all over again, I would not change my decision to support the child or the mother. I also know now that although my capacity for support is large, I am not meant to use its full extent to the point of compromising my own health and wellbeing.

Since that time I have learned to evaluate the agencies where I am considering working to see if their policies are congruent with my health and self-care. I continue to exercise regularly and am unwilling to overextend myself or compromise my wellbeing. I now live in another state and have various positions which have up until now met my needs. I periodically look to adjust my way of working to meet my changing needs as I continue to grow and learn what it means to be a change agent and an embodied being.

GRACE'S STORY

The following is a personal testimony from Grace, whose challenges, decisions, and changes she made illustrate so many of the symptoms and challenges of compassion fatigue. Having worked in both child safety and workforce investment, Grace is not only a professional service provider, she is also a family caregiver. She also shares the positive outcomes that can occur when we learn the importance of self-care and intentionally restructure our life for our own well-being.

Compassion Fatigue. That term was not in my vocabulary before I met Beverly Kyer. But before that day was over, I had so many aha moments that it became a term I shall never forget. It explained so much. At one point in the last 20 years I honestly thought that I was going crazy–or at the very least had early onset Alzheimer's. I got into social work because I am a goal-oriented person and I like helping people set goals and make changes in their lives. For more than thirty years I have been a social worker, helping the 'hard to serve.' I have worked in Workforce Investment for over ten years, and now I work for the Department of Child Safety. When I was with Workforce Investment, I have helped many people correct their paths, make good choices, and improve their lives. I have heard many tragic stories, and many times I watched those I worked with struggle within their broken relationships and broken lives, and I ached with them when they settled for less than the success that we had planned. But, I really felt that I was making a difference. During that same time I went through deceit and betrayal in my own personal life, resulting in a divorce. I worked three jobs as a single parent for several years then met and married a wonderful man with five children. We had eight children between us and I can honestly say that managing our blended family was the most challenging job I have ever done. Hands down, it was also the most rewarding, but there was never ending drama and challenges as our children navigated their adolescence, grew up, and began their own families. The emotional investment never ended, and the long days and nights ran together, blurring work, church, and family responsibilities. After our children were raised, we took in my mother-in-law and cared for her nearly eight years.

So when did I realize that the way I lived was taking a toll on my life? I realized it only in hindsight. I struggled with insomnia, mood swings, hormone imbalances, and a variety of chronic sinus problems and colds. But the greatest casualty by far was my short term memory. I recall with horror the day I couldn't remember my home phone number. This lasted not for a few moments, but for several days. Finally, I could recall it without looking it up. Many mornings I would set an appointment for the same afternoon, but when afternoon came, the appointment would pass without a thought from me. I cannot count how many wedding receptions, church dinners, meetings, and conference calls I missed because I forgot them. I was functioning at a high level in so many arenas that very few noticed all the things I forgot, but I knew a many of the plates I should have kept spinning were falling all around me. I fought silently with this for at least ten years, too embarrassed to admit to my husband or my co-workers that I forgot simple things, like what street the family I had visited ten times was on or how to operate the VCR remote. I would make myself secret notes so I could prompt myself through repetitive tasks.

Then my body began to betray me. I injured myself many times: sprained ankles, ruptured discs in my back and then neck, and torn rotator cuffs, first in one shoulder and then the other. I have had reparative surgeries four times and physical therapy at least eight times for these injuries. In time, the injuries became more serious because I could no longer heal well: injured tendons calcified and arthritis plagued my joints. Accommodating one injury would exacerbate another. I ate to comfort myself and gained weight, and then I told myself that I had so many blessings I should be happy. But I was not happy; I was scared to death and always exhausted.

I can honestly say I did not make the connection between the emotional demands I placed on myself and my physical symptoms until I heard Beverly speak about Compassion Fatigue Syndrome. It was such a relief to realize I was not going crazy and that my symptoms and suffering weren't just part of getting old. I sat down and reviewed all that I learned and made a plan. It began with recognition and acceptance, then a few steps at a time to triage the activities that created a drain and adjust them or balance them with activities that would recharge my batteries. I accepted a much less stressful job, despite the lower pay, so I could leave work at work. I let go of many betrayals and issues that were weighing me down, and I forgave myself for not being perfect. I began playing beautiful instrumental music to go to sleep, and I moved my bedtime an hour earlier. I practiced at work memorizing numbers in sequence–first only three, now I can handle seven. I admitted my memory problem to my husband and now he helps me remember the calendar. I write everything down and throw the sticky notes away when it is safe to do so. I am not forgetting as much now as I was only a year ago.

My husband and I are also on a healthy eating kick that I really enjoy. It's not too structured, so there is no built-in guilt. I eat smart: as much protein as carbohydrates, but in smaller portions than before. I skip dessert, except an occasional treat for lunch. We don't eat late at night, but I drink vitamin water or something with no calories that tastes a little sweet. I snack on nuts. I like the food; I am not hungry, and I have lost 35 pounds in the last year, which is halfway to my realistic goal. I have not found time to read, but I have found time to listen to music and to work out five times a week. I feel more in control and less stressed than I have in many years. This seems to be an ongoing battle, though. My barometer for too much stress is still my memory. And when I occasionally let myself get overloaded I still have a memory loss flare up. I still have to tell myself NO when I start to volunteer for everything that needs to get done, whether at work or church. I can tell when it is time to go out to eat and watch a movie with my husband instead of meeting some arbitrary deadline for getting the dishes or laundry done. I feel like I have my life back, with all its wonderful freckles and faults. And last but not least, I feel like I have some control over the stress level in my life.

Author's note: Like many in my position, I did not tell my immediate family of my struggles: my exhaustion, clumsiness; accident proneness, insomnia, and acute episodes of grief and fear regarding my patients and clients. I wanted them each to see me as supermom and super wife as I lovingly expended energies I did not have to care for them. This was quite detrimental to my physical and emotional health. Following the advice of others wiser than myself, I finally confessed that I was struggling. My children, the wonderful human beings that they are, immediately assumed more responsibilities, which was a great relief to me. My adopted daughter even took responsibility to check in on me from across country, always admonishing me to take better care of myself. My youngest son, who also works in child welfare, reminds me constantly to slow down and to decompress (his favorite term) and my then-husband took on most of the food preparation and cooking. He lovingly reminded me daily to be good to myself.

Now here is an interesting revelation. My then-husband, the man in my life who knew me well, had noticed all along that I was struggling. He feared that had he pointed this out earlier, I may have taken offense, thinking that he saw me as weak and incapable. He was very relieved that I was able to open up and be honest with him and allow him to help me more.

DAVID'S STORY

David is a remarkable man I met who early on wisely decided to take care of himself by consistently unwinding and recharging himself. I am especially pleased that he shared his story as he speaks to men who too often find it difficult to express their struggles and challenges in this trauma-inducing work. David is quite candid and insightful about what needed be done for his own self-care and why. His story also speaks to women who find it particularly difficult to stop, rest, and unwind. David illustrates a common range of negative scenarios affecting the personal and professional lives of workers in the helping professions.

I have worked in social services since 1999. Right out of college I worked as a counselor in a level 12 group home. I was thrown right into restraints, and dealing with the issues of what we then called SED (severely emotionally disturbed) teens. Right away, I made friends among my colleagues and hung out with many of them outside of work. I was young, so yes we partied and had a great time. The details are not important, but the unwinding was important. And for the men who managed or succeeded at staying around in this traumatic field, the unwinding was firmly part of their lives. I worked there for a year and loved the job.

As my career took me to other places, I noticed that unwinding didn't seem as important to other colleagues. I hurt my knee in 2001. My life prior to that was filled with a lot of athletic activity. I got back into social services working at a recovery program in West Oakland. I also gained part-time employment at the County Receiving home; a first stop for kids 11 years and older who were removed from their homes due to abuse. We supervised and helped these shocked and scared youth until placement was found.

As I worked these two jobs I was also planning my first wedding. This time was the most stressful of my life. Concurrently, I lost a dear friend to gun violence in Atlanta. I lost a client to HIV and another one to domestic violence retaliation between a drug addicted couple, and a young man was murdered outside my office—a random killing due to the dangerous area where we worked. I needed a lot of counseling help with my feelings around these tragedies. These events still stick with me and I know that I must process them when they float to the surface. My then-fiancé was unable to understand and be supportive to the stress manifesting in me and so my engagement fell apart. This event too was a major stressor.

How did I remain sane? I think it's because I had my "unwinds" in place: video games, social gatherings with loved ones, and coaching little league baseball, to name just a few. I always made time for these activities during stressful times, and these activities helped me remain centered and kept me from burning out on the job.

The substance recovery field is different from other caregiving fields because many of the men who work there are in recovery themselves. For that reason, finding wholesome activities that allow these men to unwind after work is difficult. Often, their past definition of fun was attached to addicting or illicit activities, making any inappropriate use of their idle time compromise their recovery. I actually saw this happen more than once. Watching a colleague self-destruct is as traumatic as watching a family member self-destruct.

I left the field for a short while, from 2006-2007, to pursue a new opportunity in the corporate world that had opened up and then closed almost as quickly. After that, I landed the job that I have now as a senior case manager working with families who are suffering due to displacement and drug addicted biological parents and grandparents. I help manage the challenging behaviors of traumatically distressed grandchildren. I have been at this job for the longest I have ever held a single position. I think it has to do with how more mindful I am about the things that keep my stress levels low, and what works.

My advice to all caregivers is to find the things make you happy (in your off-hours) and simply DO them, and don't let anyone tell you that you don't deserve the things that you enjoy doing.

SINBAD'S STORY

Sinbad shares his story of work stressors and how he takes care of himself. He shares too his unique insights on his self-caring strategies for himself his colleagues.

I have been employed for over 20 plus years with the Department of Corrections Division of Juvenile Justice where I work with incarcerated young men and young women, ages 14 to 25. Most of these young men and women have committed felonies. I am responsible for safety and security while also providing crisis intervention and counseling.

Some of the stress comes from the consistent conflicts between middle and upper management. Other stress comes from dealing with a population that's used to living in highly reactive and negative ways. I sometimes feel that as an officer my hands are tied as to what I can do to alleviate some of the stressors. Much of my challenge comes from separating the security side of my role from the rehabilitation side. Both roles are so needed by the youth, but many times these two sides conflict. And when this happens it hurts the youth as well as service providers.

Over the years on the job, I have seen many of my peers become consumed in this line of work. They start out being one person and totally transform into another. I believe this is because they don't have an outlet where they can discharge their stress and refuel.

Early on, I developed habits and outside activities to help me reduce the risk of compassion fatigue. I also strive to create a balance in my life by being involved with outside activities working with the same age group but in more positive settings. For instance, I coach college football and I mentor youth, and both of these pursuits balance me and lift my spirits and act to counterbalance the negative issues I face on the job each day.

I seek and love opportunities to experience more positive outcomes for youth who have experienced damaging and traumatic life orientations. I indulge in my favorite hobbies; golf, photography, fun family time, entertainment, and creative arts activities. I believe this has kept me inspired and has sustained my morale.

CHAPTER 7:
MORE STORIES FROM THE FIELD

Are you living or just existing?

—Tyler Perry

In this chapter, we continue looking at case studies. The first is from a nurse, Lois, who tells us about her compassion fatigue. And in our second story, we meet a woman who was a first responder and has had to deal with the effects of post-traumatic stress disorder (PTSD) and compassion fatigue following her experiences. Both of these women have generously agreed to share their stories with us here.

LOIS'S STORY

As a nurse, Lois served on the front lines of caregiving and has the stories to prove it. She also developed compassion fatigue as a result of her work and the way she managed her life outside work. Her tale is both instructive and cautionary.

As a nurse, my compassion fatigue didn't happen overnight. It happened over the course of a career. I remember driving into the parking lot of S Ward, the psychiatric unit where I worked. Every day I performed the same ritual as I pulled down the curtain over my personal life and transformed into my professional super nurse persona, much like Clark Kent stepping into a phone booth. I was proud to be leaving my baggage at the door because isn't that what superheroes are supposed to do? My professional self had always been confident, capable, and fearless. I broke up fights, advocated for patients' rights, stayed late listening to problems, and walked the halls as a paragon of the compassionate and righteous caregiver. I was numb in my personal life, however; through deaths, divorce, children, and friends, I was asleep through most of it. I did not realize that the demands of work left me empty, without much else to give at home. Work was where I poured all of my energy into the intense needs of others, and I did that job well.

When I became addicted to pain pills after some surgery that I had, my boundaries all blurred. The personal and professional crashed into each other daily. I went to work late and hungover and left early, and I often fell asleep at the desk dreaming of my next dose of inner soothing. Despite all this, I still believed I was doing my best work, and nobody ever challenged me. I was a caregiver, helping others, but where was the support for me when I needed help? I kept my struggles private. At home, I was isolated, and I suffered in silence. I overcompensated at work, convinced that I was the only one who cared, the lone warrior who could single-handedly fix everyone else's broken lives.

Eventually, each client I helped out started to take a toll on my psyche. There was Thomas, a 30-year-old man with schizophrenia, who buried his urine in jars in his yard and dressed like the 16-year-old girls whose magazine photos he collected. The treatment team decided to withhold the truth from Thomas that he was going to a long term facility the next day. He thought he would be returning home. I was the last nurse to work with him before discharge and

I participated in the lie. This has haunted me for 20 years. Thomas never spoke to me again.

And then there was Lisa, an intelligent and educated woman who fell apart after a brutal attack. She came to me sobbing with a three-day eviction notice from her mobile home park after she adopted a pet pit-bull. I spent 45 minutes on hold connecting her with legal aid, and spent years writing letters, giving depositions, and testimony on her behalf. The mobile home park spent hundreds of thousands of dollars to make an example of her and they won in court. We were both devastated, but she moved on. I was finding it increasingly difficult to reconcile my illusion of super nurse with the person I had become. I was unknowingly struggling with compassion fatigue, and as a result, I now felt like a failure in both my personal and professional lives.

For the last four years I have been stepping slowly through the fires of recovery and therapy. The most difficult part of my recovery has been accepting my human limitations. Now, when I come to work, I no longer step behind an imaginary curtain to transform into a supernurse. The person you see at work is the same person everywhere I go, whether at home, with my friends, with my children, or at the grocery store. She is always present, compassionate, and flawed, sometimes confident and sometimes afraid, sometimes taking on too much, and sometimes leaving things for the next shift. The recovering addict in me will always want more painkillers, while the recovering supernurse in me will always put others first. Recovery from drug addiction and having a super nurse complex is a lifelong process, and I will probably always struggle with these challenges. Now there is another voice inside me that reminds me every day that who I am and what I do are enough. When I feel I can't handle these challenges on my own,

I now have friends to talk to, meetings to attend, and the grateful understanding that the burden is not mine alone to carry.

ANNE'S STORY

My first EMS call as an EMT left me stunned.

As a rookie firefighter/EMT in a career fire department, the senior person and I responded to a call for what's known as a one down. We found a middle aged man lying across his front door threshold, not breathing but with a heartbeat. I performed my first CPR efforts, yet the man died.

This mid-forties man, a contributing member of society and father, husband, and worker was dead. I felt responsible for his death, and I acutely experienced the loss his death left in the world.

I finished the 24-hour shift, went home, and woke up the next morning feeling horrid guilt. I didn't know what to do so I called the fire house and spoke with the officer in charge that day, who told me you can't win them all and to move on.

I was 25 years old and thought I was invincible, but this experience left me knowing that although I loved the work and thrived in the team atmosphere, possessed the demanding critical thinking skills and the love and ability to help people, my sensitivity was going to cause me problems in this career.

As the years passed, I ran call after call, being exposed to every type of incident imaginable: suicide by gunshot, hanging, car exhaust, knife, and pills, and I saw drownings, burnt bodies, hazardous material spills, domestic violence, nursing care injuries, live births, house and commercial fires, dump fires, airplane wrecks, cars into houses, cars into people, cars over embankments, motorcycle wrecks, and shootings. I went on so many CPR calls I lost track, dealt with mentally ill patients, heart attacks, strokes, diabetic comas, each incident etching its toll on my psyche.

As my career progressed, I obtained my BS in Fire Science so I could become a Fire Chief, and I earned certifications in confined space, trench, high angle, swift water, and underwater rescue. I joined specialty teams such as the Federal Emergency Management Agency (FEMA) and the National Association of Search & Rescue (NASAR), earning the titles of Plans Officer and Technical Specialist, exposing me to more interesting and critical calls like 20-foot deep trench collapses requiring engineers to resolve them, workers trapped in highway asphalt machines requiring flight surgeons to extract them, and hurricanes on the Eastern seaboard and the Caribbean requiring search dogs and doctors to locate and treat the missing.

I began to not need to be first in on calls, volunteering instead to take less exciting positions in the command post, letting more morbid co-workers take the task of picking up body parts after a plane wreck and walking away when they would describe the scene.

And then the Oklahoma City bombing happened. My FEMA search & rescue team and I were flown to the scene, and I spent two days recording the removal of body parts of adults and children, forever leaving me profoundly emotionally scarred in a way I didn't understand at the time–I just knew I wasn't right anymore, feeling unstable, lost, and alone. I was then transferred to the command post where bodies were now numbers on paper instead of in my face, but then I was isolated from my peers, creating a huge void of support and comfort. Everything felt surreal.

This was in the days before cell phones, and they provided the rescuers with phone banks to call home, but I couldn't figure out how to explain to my family what was happening at the site or to me. Nor did I wish to poison them with stories of horror and strain. After working 13+ hour shifts in a bombed building of dust, bodies, hard concrete, and emotionally exhausting effort, eating, cleaning up, and sleeping, I didn't have the energy to try and sound chipper and upbeat, so I didn't call home. Concerned, my family called my officers who, instead of asking why I wasn't calling home, ordered me to call home, which further drained my energies.

Eight days after the bombing, I was the officer in charge at a basement house fire that was fueled by propane. Basement fires are known to be "widow makers" because floors collapse and kill rescuers, so the pressure was on! Being the officer in charge means you're in charge of orchestrating personnel, equipment, the injured, and the public, so it's incredibly nerve-wracking. On top of that, it was 1996 and I was a newly promoted officer and a woman working in a career (as opposed to volunteer) fire department, making it even more nerve-wracking. Add to that the ever-present need to perform well and keep everyone on your shift safe from harm.

Everything went wrong on that house fire: the driver didn't hear me tell him where the fire hydrant was so we didn't lay out our water supply line, the firefighter took off before I could give him instructions, volunteers arrived unexpectedly and wanted to know what to do, my fire glove was missing, the radio was on the wrong channel, the nozzle wasn't working properly, I fell down the stairs injuring my legs, the firefighter fell down the stairs damaging his breathing tank, and the hose line burnt through and we lost water. But there's more: the windows in the basement were tiny and could not fit a human escape, there was too much radio traffic to send out a call that we were trapped and needed to be rescued, the propane was feeding the fire making it burn hot and furious, both firefighters were running out of air, and the basement was completely black and the heat had banked down. All I could think was WE ARE TRAPPED AND WE ARE GOING TO DIE BY FIRE.

Later, after the fire was out, after my firefighter was on his way to the hospital, after the rehab personnel determined I was physically fit to be released, after I went to the canteen and scarfed cookies, after the house was pulled apart for lurking hot spots, after the equipment was cleaned and returned to service, after the reports were completed and filed, and after the debriefing, it was time for me to pay the emotional piper. Except this time the piper wanted more than I had to give. I was broken even more than before, and now my ability to disassociate, process, and return to center utterly failed me. The Oklahoma City bombing and the house fire together had entirely unnerved me, and I when I woke up the next morning, I was not right. And I had no way to get right, no one to call, and nowhere to go.

What followed was three long, miserable years of nightmares, sleep walking, flash backs, depression medication, violet nighttime terrors, and psychotherapy 3-4 times a week. In that time I found religion. From that time forward I avoided fire houses, fire engines, uniforms, sirens, dead animals in the road, and meat at the store. I had lost my career and I was unable to leave the house, staying in the closet because it was safer. I slept 20 hours a day, ate junk carbs and became obese, and suffered severe anxiety and extreme emotional upheavals, but the worst, most damaging and painful aspect was that my peers didn't call me. The isolation and rejection of my peers and the loss of my career was the most painful experience, and it played into my PTSD.

Being a firefighter means NEVER showing weakness in the form of emotion, and my peers didn't want to be associated with anything emotional. Reaching out to me meant exposing themselves to my emotional weakness, a contamination they could never live down. And frankly, if I hadn't had my PTSD experience, I wouldn't know what a person in my position was going through, what to say to them, or how to be there for them, and I would have been in the same tenuous position of my peers, not wanting to expose myself to an emotional peer because my reputation as a competent fire officer mattered more.

It took me three years to get through the initial wave of PTSD. Then followed YEARS of adjusting, learning, and accepting the new normal, testing my emotional capacity for daily tasks, discovering what made the day better and what created havoc, withdrawing from depression drugs and decreasing my therapy, and losing weight and learning to eat well again. I accepted that I was 32 years old and didn't have a career anymore and that I wasn't the invincible, powerful, intelligent career woman I used to be.

During this time, I learned I could do one outside task a day, like get the car oil changed or go to the grocery store, and that this one task exacted a huge emotional toll, so I needed to be prepared to nurture myself afterwards. My anxiety was generalized and debilitating. I would wake up with panic attacks with my heart racing at 200 beats per minute and no known way to change it, although I spent hundreds of dollars trying alternative therapies, essential oils, teas, anything to stop the craziness. Making it through the day was itself a challenge, much less holding a full time job! I tackled smaller challenges like taking one college class or refinishing a dresser. I forced myself out of the house by getting my SCUBA certification and then helping teach it a few days a week. And I learned, over many years, that I could do a little more, and a little more.

And then, 16 years later, after acupuncture, emotional freedom technique (EFT), eye movement desensitization and reprocessing (EMDR), more therapy, energy work, and attempts to mildly medicate myself with alcohol and pot, my romantic partner fell three stories when the construction scaffolding he was working on collapsed under him. I was his only rescuer since we were at a house on a semi-remote mountain top with no close neighbors and no cellular phone service available. After we left the hospital and I carried his 200 pound broken body up a flight of stairs and nursed him when he couldn't walk or care for himself for three weeks, I had a PTSD relapse.

I went to the local Veterans Clinic for help, which has excellent PTSD programs. I underwent two 12-week imaginal sessions, which entailed an incredibly painful reopening of the memory box and reliving and exploring every aspect of the original exposure. In these sessions I had to daily and forcefully expose myself to my stress triggers, like seeing the meat department at a grocery store. While I still can't buy, cook, or eat meat, I can now tolerate seeing raw meat at the store or a dead animal in the road. I no longer have severe meltdowns when an emergency vehicle blasts by, only a well-ingrained emotional upheaval that is manageable. I discovered my nightly nightmare of struggle is of being trapped in the basement fire where it is hot, dark, I cannot get out and I am going to die. While I may still awake to disheveled sheets, they are no longer ripped and torn.

After 19 years of high anxiety and another 12-week VA course in Acceptance and Commitment Therapy (ACT), I could now tolerate going to 5-7 grocery stores a day, which is up from 1-2 stores a day. I still can't hold down a full time job, but I can manage an easy, on call, as needed, low stress, part time sales position a few days a week.

I still isolate myself from activities I used to enjoy but now sap my energy. I no longer volunteer in soup kitchens or as a hospice respite worker, foster animals, or help with the children in church. I simply do not have the reserves to be the caregiver I used to be, and I love and forgive myself anyway.

PTSD has wreaked havoc on my love life and friendships as well. Most people cannot comprehend my emotional limitations and expect me to just "get over it." Therefore, most people, even my dearest friends, do not know I have PTSD. I don't wish to be judged; I do not want to explain myself, again and again. I don't want pity; instead, I seek to be perceived and treated as a normal person.

When I am in a romantic relationship I HAVE to share what has happened to me: I have to explain. I have to try to articulate, because they cannot understand how life is for me now, how they can help and hinder me, that I need to call a timeout sometimes and that they need to respect that, and that I don't have the emotional capacity of a non-injured person. My emotional battery doesn't have much capacity, so everything has to be doled out in metered doses.

Is PTSD compassion fatigue? That is for the professionals to decide. I do know that I am extremely blessed to have a lifetime pension for my PTSD injury so I can live paycheck to paycheck on disability and not have to worry about being homeless or hungry, but I can't afford the normal luxuries, like a vacation or a nice car, in my life either. After finding my once-in-a-lifetime career, I lost it and then spent the majority of this lifetime surviving the injury. I would much rather have been able to keep working and retain my career, but my PTSD has changed that. I live each day with gratitude for the recovery I have made, and continue to make, and I try to learn a lesson from each experience.

I would like to point out that Anne suffered and collapsed from both direct PTSD and secondary traumatic stress disorders. Please note that many of you in the workforce not only experience the impacts of compassion fatigue, but you also experience personal injuries and direct threats to your physical safety and life. It is critically important that you too get help distinguishing and treating both your PTSD and your secondary traumatic experiences.

CHAPTER 8:
TREATMENT

Failures and fears are the part of the journey we call life. Don't let them stop you or derail you from your chosen path.

—Debasish Mridha

If you, or someone you work with, have compassion fatigue, the next step should be some kind of treatment. But how should this be done? What steps you should take? These are great questions, and I'll try to answer them in this chapter. And as part of answering them, I'd like to pick up my story where we left off in Chapter 2.

MY STORY, CONTINUED

After that initial episode, my first doctor misdiagnosed me with bronchial asthma. I didn't agree with her because I never had allergies or any other respiratory conditions. Further, I told her that I always worked in my garden, weeding and cutting the grass, with no breathing distress. She still gave me an inhaler and some prednisone, which did provide me some immediate yet temporary breathing relief.

But as I was checking out at the clinic's reception desk, my improved breathing took a nosedive. My chest felt tight, I felt nauseous and weak, and my legs couldn't hold me up. The staff helped me back to the treatment room and gave me a massive dose of prednisone and another air treatment. After I stabilized, I could breathe easier. I was sent home with a nebulizer. I drove myself.

Once home, I could do little more than sit in my recliner. I was exhausted and didn't dare lie down. I felt a suffocating and crushing pressure on my chest if I wasn't sitting upright, so I slept at night in the recliner. I called my doctor several times over the next three days to report that I felt only momentary relief after using the inhaler. Beyond that, I did not think it was working for me. After I made several calls, my doctor, in her frustration, told me that if it would make me feel better I could take a cardiac stress test. Maybe the asthma (she was still insisting I had Asthma) is cardiac in nature, she told me.

The cardiologist who oversaw the stress test was energetic and enthusiastic and put me at ease with his humor. The treadmill part of the test was very exhausting, but I got through it. When I laid down on the cot he looked at the monitor and exclaimed: "That asthma diagnosis is a big red herring; your heart muscles do not want to pump, young lady." He helped me sit up and showed me the monitor. I could see in the monitor that my heart very slowly and partially contracted and then hesitated before relaxing only partially. To my untrained eyes it looked as if my heart would stop at any second. I was seeing my own mortality. All at once I was scared and sad for the life I was going to lose.

I was sent home (this time driven by a friend!) and told to call my referring doctor for instructions once she reviewed the cardiac test findings. I next experienced a complete shutdown in communications. The referring doctor would not take any of my many calls. Her receptionist kept referring me back to the cardiologist, who in turn insisted I speak to my referring doctor (because she had primary responsibility for my case, he said). This went on for two long days. As if receiving a message from beyond, it suddenly occurred to me that these people were going to continue to avoid me, allowing me to die. If anyone questioned them, they could then chalk it up to my being overweight, which I was.

My doctor had failed to give me much helpful advice about my new and alarming condition, so I made two lifesaving decisions. First, I called and explained my situation to my acupuncturist who saw me within two hours and did some intensive work that reduced the backup of fluid in my lungs. This soon relieved much of the pressure on my chest. My acupuncturist also worked to improve functioning of the heart muscles over the next few days.

The second lifesaving thing that I did was to ask my employer's human resources department for authorization to go to another medical facility that specialized in cardiac care and get tested again. In other words, I asked them to authorize a second cost outlay for the same condition. This was authorized on the recommendation of a knowledgeable family friend (thank you Barbara F.!). I selected a new primary care doctor and got an immediate emergency appointment.

As I sat with my new physician during my first appointment, the first thing that struck me was how long he silently read and re-read pages of my medical history. He was clearly scanning back and forth, seeming to synthesize the information before him and making lots of notes. Occasionally, he would question me about my symptoms and then continue his intense scanning and note-taking. I thought about how thorough he was being. I seemed to really matter to this medical practitioner. After being in his office for several minutes, I had relaxed my body and sat back in the chair. I was not going to be herded through quickly to make room for the next patient waiting to be seen. He was spending as much concentrated time with me as necessary to make a sound diagnostic assessment of my condition and treatment options. This was not the standard patient in and out warehousing I had been used to. Here, I had a doctor concerned enough to try and understand what was happening to me. I felt confident that I was going to have a fighting chance to live.

When my new doctor finally spoke he stated that I was an enigma. I would remember this statement many times later as I researched the distinction between the varied presentations of heart attack or heart failure in men, women, and different ethnic groups. I did not present with the typical symptoms associated with heart failure. I did not experience the gripping chest pain or the numb left arm. I have since learned that, like me, many women from various racial groups, and some men of color, lose their lives (or come close) because their heart failure doesn't present with the typical life-threatening symptoms.

My doctor ordered various tests, again thoroughly summarizing the findings, and determined that I had restrictive cardio myopia. This is a heart chamber muscle disease that impedes the pumping of fluid in and out of my heart. The condition reduced the flow of oxygen-rich blood to my brain and body, resulting in a debilitating fatigue. It also caused a flooding of fluid in my lungs, which was the reason I needed to sit upright in a chair day and night to sleep if I didn't want to feel like a bear was sitting on my chest.

INTENSE CARDIAC REHAB, RE-PROGRAMMING AND DOWN SHIFTING

The fact that I'm writing this book means I was able to survive. And I survived only after making major changes, because now I intentionally give myself time for proper rest and recovery, and the time to talk stressful events out with someone.

I was not sure that I would live through cardiac rehab. I was so weak and prone to feeling faint while doing my exercises that I thought I would expire at any time. Each time I entered the rehab center I was attached to monitors linked to the exercise machines. I was closely supervised for each of the prescribed exercises. While I was exercising, the rehab staff watched the monitors. Countless times they had to come running to my exercise station to rescue me. The goal was to get my heart muscles to work and pump in a regulated rhythm, but during those emergencies my heart rate would speed up way beyond a normal level or drop dangerously low, creating terrifying sensations of breathlessness, weakness, loss of consciousness, and collapse. I felt very anxious most of the time because being unable to breathe and carry my weight on my legs terrified me.

For the three days a week over those three months that I was on those exercise machines, I did a lot of thinking. I thought about what I would do differently if I got to live longer. I thought about all the things I missed doing because I had been too busy and too emotionally exhausted to do them. I have talents and God-given artistic gifts that I put on the shelf while waiting for some opportune time that never seemed to come. For the past several years, I was always up to my neck in work, work, work.

I felt ashamed. I thought about people I know who live quality lives, and I questioned my life choices. Why and when did I decide that I was born solely for service to others? As I have said before, I know where I got this notion from. I loved my father dearly and watched him die much too soon. And here I was, following in his footsteps to an early grave. I did lots of reading and got lots of counseling in an effort to re-program my thinking about my life and what was left of it.

Some of my counselors have told me that I throw myself into relentless work schedules: waist high into the suffering of others so that I don't have to think about the losses I've personally experienced. To the extent that I could accept this, I decided simply to be happy, which I think is so much better than simply being content.

The first step to re-program myself was to live without a clock. I shut off the alarm and paid attention to the clock only for my rehab/medical appointments. How wonderful it is to allow your body to gently become aware of a new day. This is so much more pleasant than the jarring sounds of an alarm. It was only then that I began to gently rouse myself to full alertness before rising from my bed. When I start my day like this, I start in a state of regulated calm.

The rest of the time during those three months of rehab I slept, ate, read pleasurable books or simply daydreamed according to the needs and desires of my body, mind, and spirit. During this period I began to be aware of my spirit; I had urgings to re-engage in the arts and connect with friends just for fun. I also began to really enjoy my surrounding as I noticed features of my home and gardens as if for the very first time in a very long time. I would visit other rooms and spaces in and around my house. (E.g. my guest room, my living room, the side and back yards) I would just sit, notice and experience those environments. This may sound strange, but it seemed that I was just starting to fully appreciate and live in the home that I purchased five years prior.

I further began to dream dreams and have visions of wonderful possibilities. I became inspired to adorn and enhance those newly experienced areas of my home—just little touches purchased at the home decorating departments of Ross, T.J. Maxx, or at Burlington. I didn't want to spend a lot of money but to beautify the newly discovered areas of my home.

Infused with a creative and physical energy I had not experienced in years, I was next inspired to start a free weekly dancing school at church. I managed, designed, and choreographed weekly classes for the beautiful and talented children there who performed magnificently once a month for three solid years. This was one of the most powerful and therapeutic aspects of my healing.

After my healing began, I noticed a change in how I woke up. Now, when I awoke I would gently become aware of a new day via the sunlight filtering through my windows, sensing my body and spirit re-aligning as if I had been on an out of body trip during the night. Prior to my healing, I used to arise quickly from my bed on waking. I would then notice a slight unsteadiness in my gait and even sometimes a slight dizziness. But after I began to heal, I would lie still after waking, just for a moment, to allow my spirit to lock onto the landing station which is my body. Of course, this means that I did not allow my thoughts to hasten to action (leaping from bed) to meet the needs of the day. Instead, I took care to enjoy those moments, just a few, to be bodily aware of myself, to allow the body-spirit alignment that says I am ready to move forward into this new day.

Each morning as I gradually woke up I would immediately greet God in appreciation and gratitude for each new day and then become aware of inspirational ideas entering my mind: things to do or to try. I learned to execute things that came to me first thing in the morning. These good things have always resulted in days where I accomplished projects and key tasks with ease.

SEEKING TREATMENT

No matter what stage of compassion fatigue a direct care worker is experiencing, the trajectory of the stress hormone will create a shift in their brain chemistry, causing changes in their feelings, emotions, and behaviors. And no matter how unfit, unproductive, or uncooperative a worker may appear to be, expedient and compassionate treatment can shift the brain chemistry to a regulated, resilient and healthier state.

Treatment for compassion fatigue needs to come on a variety of fronts: via supervision, employee assistance program (EAP), team support, stress management methods, a licensed clinician, accountability partners, and one's own support community. It is only by attacking compassion fatigue on these various fronts can the sufferer's personal well-being, performance, and job satisfaction be restored.

Successful Tools, Strategies and Methods for Recovery

In this section, I want to talk about some of the strategies and tools that you can use to help you recover from compassion fatigue.

Intervention: *Where to Seek Help*

Seeking help is the smart step to take when you begin to feel yourself (or someone tells you that you are) experiencing compassion fatigue. This is the best time to deal with it since waiting for symptoms to become debilitating only prolongs the restoration of well-being and job satisfaction.

I suggest you seek help from the following sources:

- An understanding and trusted friend or family member
- Your work supervisor
- Work team members
- Your chosen accountability partners
- Professional therapists or counselors
- Spiritual advisors and counselors
- Pastoral counseling
- Employee assistance program(EAP)
- Co-workers
- Family physician
- Trauma-informed specialist
- Support group facilitators
- Certified Compassion Fatigue Specialists

Intervention: *recognizing stress within yourself*

This is an exercise to increase awareness of what is happening in our bodies during stressful events. We tend to pay attention to major traumatic events (we certainly note their impact on those we are caring for), yet we ignore the seemingly less significant events and their impact on us. As a result, we allow multiple stressors to accumulate in our mind and body, much to our detriment. In other words, we allow ourselves to become flooded with stress hormone.

Remember that your body keeps score

For this exercise, think of a minor stressor or small annoyance. This could be an interaction with a particular person, a place you have to visit, a project you're working on, or even a sound that causes slight feelings of irritation. Now make a note of the stressor in the box below.

A minor stressor in my life:

┌───┐
│   │
│   │
│   │
│   │
└───┘

Where do you physically experience this stressor?:

┌───┐
│   │
│   │
│   │
│   │
└───┘

An exercise to locate and reduce physical stress

1. Now, think deeply and try to determine where in your body the stress is experienced when you think of the situation you've just identified. Try to mentally scan your body from head to foot, noticing if any sensation results because of that stressor. This can help you understand how your body

reacts to stress, and can give you a place to start as you try to decrease physical and emotional stress.

2. Once you noticed the location and sensations such as tightness, fluttering, aches, pain, tingling, etc., place your hand over the area and imagine that you can see the actual location.

3. Next, breathe deeply and slowly as if sending breath right to the area to calm it and slow down the stress hormone. Emotion and memory get stuck in your stress areas, and in this exercise you are helping to release past histories, current triggers, and recent distressing content.

You may wish to test this the next time you face this specific stressor, and if you have the same reaction as the one you experienced today, you can be sure that this is where your body feels this stress and you can attend to the area of the body that is reactive to the trigger.

Intervention: discharging disturbing material

I want to focus now on the importance of discharging disturbing material. Memories, both positive and negative, are stored in cells throughout the body, and as I stated earlier, the body keeps score. The body remembers. During events and experiences that trigger these memories, we feel a measure of discomfort or unease. We can give meaning to the distress when the triggering factor is very evident, like when a person is being verbally hostile, or, we may not be cognizant of what is causing an inner distress.

Being unaware of what is causing inner distress often happens when we have repressed disturbing and traumatic material, but some external trigger has re-surfaced the memories stored in our bodies and this causes us to feel and behave in ways we often do not understand. Of course, this can happen with past trauma that has not been sufficiently addressed therapeutically, but it can also happen when we experience a distressing situation that resembles one that you experienced sometime earlier. You may have forgotten about the situation or not allowed yourself to think about it, but because the body remembers, it can react, creating inner distress and stirring up of our emotions.

I am alarmed when I hear caring people urge trauma victims to not think about it or to try to forget it. I am especially concerned when I hear adults deny children the opportunity to talk about the trauma they have experienced. The adults mistakenly believe that if the trauma is not talked about, the child or adult will somehow forget and be all right. It is in these scenarios, when traumatic material is not discharged, that the adult and the child in question may be plagued by a lifetime of intrusive and invasive disturbances that unconsciously shape their thinking, feelings, and behaviors. The fact is, we must discharge traumatic exposure and events.

Intervention: when you see it in colleagues

Now that you know what to look for, you will start to notice symptoms of compassion fatigue in those you work with. And when you notice that a colleague is stressed and may be experiencing compassion fatigue, make sure to balance issues of privacy with needed action. On the one hand, you need to respect a colleague's personal space and feelings, yet on the other hand, you need to be responsible to your colleague and your agency when you see them struggling to their own detriment and the detriment of others.

In many cases, simply asking a person if they are okay, may not be enough. For many reasons, struggling colleagues may answer that they are okay, when in fact they are not. When someone clearly resists your help, you can be respectfully more directive in your approach.

You can be more directive in gentle ways. If you can continue talking with your colleague, you may acknowledge that an incident occurred and that you are concerned about them. Urging your colleague to take a few minutes to step outside, relax, and process the incident may be very helpful. If they are open to your help, you can also stay with them while they do a quick body scan to locate the tension and complete a tense-to-relax exercise and/or a breathing technique to help release the tension they find.

If the impacted colleague is overwhelmed with emotion, you can gently walk them to a private space in order to process (using narrative) their emotional stress with them. If they are about to cry, encourage them to let it flow and give them time to release whatever is coming up for them. If tears come forth from you, do not restrain them, but release your distress also.

Reassure your colleague that they are not alone and that help is available. You can also share ways in which the same or a similar stressor has impacted your life, thereby letting them know how common compassion fatigue is and how it can affect all of us. Of course, be very careful here not to make this about you. Your goal is to stay with their need for help.

By helping your colleague associate the physiological sensations that accompanied the external happening (whatever was heard, seen, smelled, tasted, or felt) with the emotions that came up for them, you can help them with the release of stored negative energy from the mind and body. In this way, you can help your colleague identify their bodily stress locations and alleviate them through deep breathing and other self-regulating techniques. An insightful client of mine named Thelma defines this integrating process as "giving meaning to the alarm."

Narrative processing—getting your colleague to tell their story—is also very effective, if your colleague is amenable to it. We will discuss the narrative process more in the next section.

If your colleague is not open to your assistance, even after giving them some time to decompress, you may want to talk to your supervisor about your concerns. This is where the balance between privacy and concerned responsibility comes in. We believe it is better to take some action and get some help than to ignore a situation that may lead to continuing struggles for your colleague, your agency and the people we serve. Note: you should also follow your department's policy regarding your responsibility to report concerns to your immediate supervisor.

Interventions: the role of narrative

In traditional narrative therapy, telling your story after a traumatic event facilitates healing. After trauma, the brain is in lockdown, screaming the following messages and more: " Disaster!–Oh my God! – What the hell just happened?" "How could something like this happen?" " Was I too late?" "I didn't do enough!" "I failed!"

After a traumatic event, the brain chemistry makes it very difficult to process what actually happened in any positive terms since it is busy with the above messaging. It is very difficult or impossible to see effective moments, positive outcomes, or the fact that you may have helped your client or patient in a significant way, often times just by being present.

Experience has taught us that people operating in the helping capacity have a strong sense of responsibility for the safety and wellbeing of the person or persons who suffered direct trauma or tragedy. This places them at risk for suffering from secondary traumatic stress or compassion fatigue. The supportive interventions of coworkers, supervisors, and a team process play a powerful role in taking that healing journey with you. So remember, it is best not to go it alone.

When possible, narrative should be used immediately after an event as the stressed out worker will no doubt be carrying the heaviness of the traumatic event. Employing the principles of expressed empathy and supporting self-efficacy, the person assisting the worker experiencing compassion fatigue can ask a series of reframing and externalizing questions which will accomplish the following:

- Recollect, realize, and articulate positive aspects they may have missed or ignored
- Become motivated to take steps to move forward
- Recognize that the trauma is something that happened but it does not define them
- Transform the painful effects of the trauma on the person; lessening the impact

It is important not to sound interrogative, but rather to ask the questions in a curious manner so that the stressed person does not feel they need to explain or defend their efforts and actions. It is a natural occurrence for someone experiencing compassion fatigue to perceive they are being judged post crisis. Instead, they should be helped to realize that their efforts were appreciated and helped in many ways. Questions should challenge negative conceptions thus promoting a somewhat more uplifting and hopeful end to the story.

Here are a few examples of statements and questions you can use to help the secondarily wounded:

- Did you realize that_____ knew you would not give up on them?
- Are you aware that most people would not have handled this situation as well as you did?
- You and _____ accomplished so much together. What did he/she like the most?
- I would like to hear some of the special times/sayings_____you shared
- Tell me some of the things he/she said that helped you remember the good experiences?
- What would you like to do next for _____
- What will help you now?

Intervention: some personal examples

Another way to use narrative as an intervention is as a person supporting/helping, you point out positive aspects of the stressed out co-worker's experience. In some ways as you'll see, this is lending light in a dark situation.

An example of this is when a young child, with whom I had worked closely for some years died as I sat next to him and held him. A supportive and insightful coworker asked if the grandmother was present at the time of the child's death. When I answered yes, my coworker then stated you know Mrs._____ could always count on you being there for her. You were there by her side during perhaps the most difficult times of her life. She would have felt hurt and alone so much more had you not been there to share the grief with her.

My colleague's comments shined some light through the crushing dark space I was in and eased some of the pain I felt. From there, after a few more of her open-ended and externalizing questions, it was possible for me to tell my story about various experiences with the child. Given the greatness of the pain I felt for this and many other children who had died on my caseload, I was not able to open up—I was choked up tightly in my chest and throat—without her first reframing the tragedy for me. I needed her to start the narrative for me, prompting me to continue. When I started telling the story my healing process began, enabling me to resume responsibilities quickly to other patients, parents, and coworkers.

In another example, I worked in a psychiatric day hospital. One of my patients in our day treatment program for US Military Veterans committed suicide. I was overwhelmed with grief complicated by guilt and shame. I felt completely responsible for not having seen this coming and stopping this tragedy. There seemed to be a huge crushing boulder on my chest. The program director, a psychiatrist, noticed my silence and manner, sat down in front of me, looked into my eyes and said Mr._____ made sure you did not know his plans because he did not want you to stop him. He (my patient) hung in as long as he did because he enjoyed talking to you. In the end, he could no longer tolerate the rest of his life, yet he very much benefited from your presence for a good while.

The sorrow I felt for a precious fragile life lost, and in such a horrific manner, is something I would contend with for a very long time, but the guilt and shame I was also struggling with was greatly alleviated because of what the Psychiatrist did for me. Going forward, I was able to share stories of past conversations with him when supportive coworkers asked me questions like: "He often laughed when he was talking to you. What was your work experience like with Mr._____?" "What were some of the topics you two shared that put him at ease and made him smile?" I began telling my story, not just the painful end-point, but the beginning and middle, which helped make it possible for me to move forward. This service to vulnerable US military veterans was then my mission.

Intervention: building a team of accountability partners

The most important and startling revelation for me as I began to research compassion fatigue (after my second bout of heart failure), was that I need accountability partners to help save me from myself. Just as our work is best done as a team, we can best manage how we experience the sufferings and traumas of others as a team. I found that caregivers who are the most successful in experiencing healthier, balanced, and happier lives and job satisfaction have people close around them for camaraderie and support. So, if you want to treat and avoid compassion fatigue, you need to develop a community of close people who are able to support you, listen and understand you and what you do (to the extent that they can), and enjoy lots of down time, relaxation, laughter, and fun with you. The people most at risk for the pitfalls of compassion fatigue are those that lack this support network.

In your non-work life, you may be surrounded by people in your family and social circle who need you to be okay and energized, so that you are always available for them. While they may love you, they also may find your fatigued or stressed out states intolerable.

They may lack understanding and respect for your work and its mission. I have had people close to me say "I don't even know why you do that type of work. You could be doing _____ or _____and getting paid a whole lot better."

These people can be an additional drain on your personal and professional energies. While many of us have these people in our lives and it is highly probable that we love them and will continue to interact with them, unless they can learn to view your work and your needs differently, they are not capable of being your therapeutic community. In short, you need to broaden your support network: you need more people.

I'm reminded of movies where I have seen fireman entering life-threatening situations together. One or more of them may stumble, get trapped, and be in jeopardy. They seem to always quote this statement "no one leaves one." They link safety belts or hands together to form a safety net, making sure that each man is connected and that no one is lost or forgotten. By working as a team to ensure each other's safety, they can maintain their intense mental focus on rescuing civilians. Connecting lifelines and hands is a physical action, but it comes from a place in the heart, to always remain connected in every risky situation. I strongly suggest that each of us in the helping professions adopt that same team spirit. I suggest that we consider operating as "loving meddlers" as we journey through this challenging and highly stressful work.

A team think tank to support coworkers with compassion fatigue

If you haven't already, form a team at work of accountability partners whose goal will be to not only support those on the team who are showing signs of compassion fatigue but also help them overcome their natural defensiveness that can come from being very stressed out and stuck.

The team starts out by giving positive feedback and pointing out what is working well, and can be built on. Then the team shares ideas and suggestions that may be beneficial, given the circumstances. This is done in a supportive manner that gently helps the worker who is stuck be able to expand their perspective and see other possibilities for addressing the current situation. I call this "team think tank."

I am certain you already have various methods for this type of support, but I do wish to emphasize the importance of people in the helping professions having "their people" and "their therapeutic community" to avoid the risk of feeling alone and isolated in work struggles.

Remember, the same signs and symptoms of compassion fatigue you notice in others can affect you as well. And as we are usually the last people to recognize emotional and behavioral changes in ourselves, this is where accountability partners play an important role. These partners can notice symptoms in you that indicate when you are beginning to be overwhelmed.

INTERVENTION: COGNITIVE RESTRUCTURING

Cognitive behavioral interventions help us see the relationship between our thoughts, feelings, and actions. By analyzing our thought processes, we are able to isolate negative, extreme, and unrealistic patterns of thought, thereby reducing stressful feelings and changing our behaviors (Meichenbaum 1975/Bandura 1977/

Beck 1976). Cognitive behavioral interventions can also minimize the distress that accompanies compassion fatigue, leading you to a calmer inner dialogue. Just like our clients, we can benefit from self-exploration that can come from cognitive restructuring. Follow the steps outlined below to conduct your own cognitive restructuring.

Step one: identify the stressor

The first step is to identify the situation that causes you stress. You can do this by asking yourself the following questions:

- Is it a particular client who comes in for an appointment?
- Is it seeing the name of a particular client on your appointment calendar when you come into work in the morning?
- Is it a disturbing phone call, or even seeing the name on the caller ID on your phone when a difficult client calls? Or is it the situation they are painfully ensconced in?
- Is it a sudden crisis or the need for an emergency response?
- Is it caused by escalating clients/patients, receiving bad news, contentious work related meetings, physical altercations in an institution, or some other recurring incident?

Step two: ground yourself

The next step in the process is to ground yourself so that you are not overwhelmed by feelings that occur when you think about the stressors. This can be done with breathing techniques, which will be described in detail later on in the book, and with relaxation techniques, both mental and physical/muscular.

Examine thinking patterns

After grounding, it is helpful to look at your thinking patterns during and after the stressors. In other words, you want to ask yourself what you are saying in your head that adds to your stress. Many times we get stuck in the following mental dialogues: "oh isn't it awful," or "this is not going to turn out good at all," or "the stuff is about to hit the wall now," etc. We often replay these mental dialogues over and over in our thoughts as if by thinking about it repetitively, we can somehow magically create a different outcome.

Many times we engage in "distorted thinking" patterns as defined by David Burns (1999). By identifying the following patterns, you can help yourself and coworkers when working to decrease stress.

All or Nothing Thinking–seeing life in black-and-white categories rather than shades of gray.

Overgeneralization–Seeing a single negative event as a never ending pattern of defeat.

Mental Filter–picking out a single negative defeat and dwelling on it exclusively so that everything in life looks bleak.

Disqualifying the Positive–dismissing positive experiences to maintain negativity, even if inconsistent with your experience. For example the infamous: "but" statement that extinguishes the previous "positive-possibility" statements.

Jumping to Conclusions–making a negative interpretation of an event even though there are no definite facts that convincingly support your conclusion.

This can be seen in both the following:

1. Mind reading–assuming negative thinking of someone else without checking to make sure you are accurate.
2. Fortune-telling–assuming and anticipating that things will turn out badly, even though there is nothing to support that assumption.

Magnification (Catastrophizing) or Minimization–this is looking at life through a set of binoculars, either exaggerating the importance of things on one end, or inappropriately shrinking the importance by looking through the other end.

Emotional Reasoning – assuming that negative emotions necessarily reflect the way things really are.

Should Statements–believing that one "should" think or act in a particular way or some horrible consequences will follow. The emotional consequence of applying this to one's self is guilt. When it is applied to others, the result is anger, frustration, and resentment.

Labeling and Mislabeling–attaching a negative label to yourself or someone else.

Personalization–Seeing yourself as the cause for some event and/ or the emotional or behavioral reactions of someone who is in crisis even though you were not the cause.

Replacing negative thoughts

Now let's consider some ways to replace negative thoughts with less emotionally charged alternatives. you'll see that just by changing to more reasonable and realistic thoughts, you can change your internal dialogue and create a more peaceful inner world.

1. A new child on your caseload has been the victim of significant abuse and neglect by both birth parents.

   Negative thought: This child has no one in his/her life to care for them and protect them. **Replacement thought**: I will prioritize focus on exploring and connecting with extended family relationships. There must be others who can participate in care for this child and support the family.

2. The grandmother of three biological young children on your caseload frequently misses your 10 o'clock meetings:

   Negative thought: She is really resistant to working with me. **Replacement thought**: It is no doubt very challenging for her to navigate scheduling to meet all the needs of her grandchildren, the system, and our agency. I will try to help her with this.

3. Your phone rings and you see the call is from a client who calls you much too often:

   Negative thought: He calls all the time as if I have no other clients but him.

   Replacement thought: He calls too often so I am going to give him a couple of scheduled times to call.

4. You have a client who consistently arrives late:

   Negative thought: I can't stand this guy. He is so inconsiderate.

Replacement thought: I wonder why he arrives late so frequently? Maybe it's a transportation issue or maybe his sense of time is different from mine. Maybe he wants to make me angry. I'm going to talk to him and find out what's going on and what he may need.

5. You have to make home visits in an unsafe neighborhood:

Negative thought: I am going to get hurt or robbed or both someday.

Replacement thought: I think I should go over safety procedures with my supervisor and team and review options for safety precautions.

6. You have a caseload of teenagers. Some deeply injured, and some very angry:

Negative thought: These kids can't be trusted.

Replacement thought: There are trust concerns for many of the kids on my caseload, but this does not apply to all kids.

7. A wife reports a number of incidents where she is physically abused by her husband:

Negative thought: I get so weary of domestic violence cases because women most likely will return to the violence.

Replacement thought: I will explore with her what factors make it difficult for her to move on. What is she afraid of?

Losing her life? Losing her financial security? Losing stability for her and the children? Or does she have a very strong love attachment? I will provide counseling and resources according to her expressed needs.

8. A client/patient is dying from a terminal illness:

    Negative thought: This is so horrible. They are absolutely cheated out of life.

    Replacement thought: I will work with my team, the patient/client and the family to assure dignity, comfort, support, and quality of life issues in the remaining days and months in this person's life.

9. A 30-year-old client tells you he was molested by his uncle when he was eight years old.

    Negative thought: He must hate his uncle.

    Replacement thought: I wonder how he feels about his uncle at this point in his life.

10. You work in Juvenile Hall.

    Negative thought: I'm going to get injured someday.

    Replacement thought: I think I should take another self-defense class so I don't get injured on the job.

11. You have a client who is basically a slob.

Negative thought: He shouldn't dress like that when he comes to my office.

Replacement thought: This man could use some guidance (or possibly some clothing) so he can learn to look more presentable when he meets with people.

So you can see from the examples, that it's not uncommon to have some distorted patterns of thinking when it comes to our jobs and caregiving and to then express those distortions in ways that will only increase our own stress. These are just a few examples of replacement thoughts that may be useful. I am sure you have many others in your own repertoire of mental responses for a host of unique situations.

The MOC theory

Many years ago one of my professors provided a tool that has been quite useful to help me move from distorted/negative thinking to more reasonable expectations for both myself and my clients and patients. That tool my professor gave me is called the MOC theory. MOC stands for Motivation, Opportunity, and Capacity. She taught to me view difficult client behaviors (e.g., non-compliant, aggressive, or mean-spiritedness) through the lens of MOC.

Motivation: because we know that all human beings have needs and desires such as safety, food, shelter, income, stability, happiness, dreams and aspirations, it is fair to assume that they are motivated for life to work out well for them. The challenge comes when, because of the chaos in their lives, they have varying ideas of how to make things work out. And so we all struggle about the best strategies and timelines.

Opportunity: this speaks to the many factors that can block a person's efforts to better their lives under our care. These factors may include, but are not limited to, the following: physical or mental illness, no bus fare, no gas in the car, lost car keys, no babysitter, sickness in the household, fighting or disturbances in the household, neighborhood threats, night blindness, fear, overcommitted scheduling, legal pressures, and competing demands with other social agencies, etc.

Of course, we need to understand these factors and work with our clients to mobilize alternative options so that we can have compliance and cooperation in our working relationships.

Capacity: this speaks to how people have uniquely learned to survive utilizing their own strengths and coping skills. Their capacity will determine when they are able to take action on our recommendations and interventions. Their level of tolerance and frustrations will determine when they push back, bark, or become confrontational with us. We must recognize that this is their capacity at this painful, confusing, and difficult point in time and has nothing to do with our abilities to provide care.

It can hurt us emotionally when our clients turn on us or act out in socially unacceptable ways. By using the MOC consistently, you can eventually ease and may even prevent some of the emotional injury from your patients and clients. Try to recognize that undesirable behaviors on their part are the direct result of their personal struggles and tragedies.

One caveat: another professor, when preparing us for a particularly challenging patient population (veterans suffering with posttraumatic stress disorders), suggested that we always consider that "all people are bewildered, until proven guilty." he believed that "their actions and behaviors are a result of their suffering and pain." He encouraged us to look past this and see our clients, and to do our very best to help in a respectful manner.

Sample

You are stressed when the parent of a traumatized child who was again incarcerated for acting out behavior is blaming you for not having done enough to prevent his or her behavior.

Trigger: you receive a call from a screaming parent who is blaming you and demanding that you get to juvenile hall immediately and fix the situation.

Your automatic thoughts: I hate when she blames me for her child's behavior when in fact she should have been in better control of her own child.

Your automatic behavior: anger, avoidance, non-supportive conversation (refusing to say anything encouraging or empathetic), and resentment.

Now let's re-think this trigger, but this time I will try to list behaviors and thoughts that are intentional, mindful, and less stress provoking. In this way, the above reactions could be replaced with the following:

Your intentional thoughts: she is really in pain and she is really afraid for her child and may even be feeling guilty. She wishes she could have prevented this, but I appear to be the person she believes she could turn to. She just doesn't know how to express her real feelings to me so she is projecting out of fear.

Your intentional behavior: I'll do some deep breathing while I listen to her and before I respond. I will acknowledge how upsetting this must be for her. I may point out that her child had been making some progress and that we will try to find out what may have triggered the setback. I will encourage her to talk to the probation officer or the child's attorney try to find out the court's decision, and then we will decide and plan our next steps together. If she feels she cannot talk to the probation officer or the attorney alone, I will suggest we schedule a three-way call.

Please notice I did not say that I would jump in and fix the situation. Regardless of her capacity to take responsibility, I respected her enough as a parent to redirect her thinking to *shared action* in this situation. Equal to my concern for the parent and the child in this particular type of scenario, I protected my own boundaries by not heaping on an unfair and unrealistic set of expectations as "the fix-it person" on myself.

Doing this exercise with several of your triggers will help you build a healthy repertoire of stress reducing inner dialogs. Practicing them over and over will eventually help you gain some inner mastery over your reactions so that you can have mindful responses rather than reactive responses to stressful events.

REVIEW

Please take a few minutes and think of work events that provoke anxiety in you. These can be anything from meeting with a particular client, supporting a terminal patient, a visit to juvenile hall for youth on your caseload who was just recently incarcerated, to a meeting where you and the client and family have reached an impasse, etc.

In the box below, write down that trigger you just thought of that causes you to begin feeling anxious.

```


```

Next, write down the automatic thoughts that enter your mind about that trigger.

```


```

Now, write down your automatic behaviors that follow that trigger and those thoughts.

```


```

Now, take a moment to gather your thoughts, and continue with the exercise, but this time write down intentional thoughts and actions.

So, in this box, write down *intentional* thoughts about that trigger.

Now, write down *intentional* behaviors that follow that trigger and thoughts.

Recap: consider your triggers and thought processes

Please review and take note of your responses. What you wrote here can help you identify future stressors and your initial thought processes and can help you prepare a more appropriate response and diffuse situations, places, or people who can act as triggers. As I did with my work and life, treating your compassion fatigue often involves changing your thinking as well as your routine.

LETTING GO

For me, letting go was a final step in my healing process. In some ways, it was the easiest step for me because I am a person of faith. Yet I left it for last because of my propensity to pick up again what I had already let go of. Having significantly anchored much of the other self-care strategies, I was better able to let go and stop worrying about things that could be managed by someone else, or situations I had little or no control over yet seemed so important for the benefit of someone in need that I would be driven to try and make it work somehow. These were no longer sacred cows. Life would go on without Beverly Kyer holding so much stuff on her shoulders.

An act of faith

Letting go is a bit like taking a free fall, and as such, it is the ultimate act of faith. This is where I let go without knowing what happens next; where do I go from here? Before I had any idea what I would do next, I literally resigned my job and was spiritually inspired to serve the same populations but in a very different way, a way that was healthier for me; a way that also fired my passions and at the same time gave me great joy. My faith assured me that how this would manifest or materialize would come to me by inspiration from God. And so I was at complete peace about this new part of my life that was just around the corner yet in the moment out of my sight. Further, I terminated many commitments that kept me overly busy without having a backup or alternate plan. My faith said to me that this is a good thing to do at this point in my life. So I left the answer to the "what's next?" question to God, and the resulting free fall felt wonderfully liberating. I gently and gloriously floated into his hands.

Embracing change

In conjunction with letting go, I also had to learn to change. And there were many issues I had to understand to ultimately embrace change:

1. I had to analyze and discard the early life messages I carried and the significance I gave them. I had to realize that many of those messages no longer applied to what I was now trying to accomplish. I had to realize the unfair and unrealistic burden they invited me to operate under. And I had to rewrite my story and include my health and wellbeing in it.

2. I needed to be honest with myself and others, that I was not doing "fine" as I usually said. I was not doing well at all. I was really struggling and needed help. For me, this was terribly hard because this was not in my vocabulary. Helpers typically do not ask for help. Certainly not I. Perhaps hardest, was to reconcile how my service as a helping professional, service that I was called to and passionate about doing, was hurting me. In the past, I could not fathom this and did not realize that I needed to take care of me while I was taking care of others. I get it now. This is hard work, painful and distressing work. As important as it is, this work comes with a price, and so I need help to do it well and take care of myself in the process.

3. I would always need accountability partners in my professional and personal life to help me, support me, remind me, and push me to take care of myself. I needed my people who, when I responded "I'm fine," would push back and say, "No! You are not."

4. I need always to discharge and transform the pain every day. For me, in addition to my special people that I can talk to, I now also have a professional clinician to help me integrate and process the traumatic material I still take in as I present to and counsel professional service providers and caregivers around the country.

SUMMING UP

As you have now hopefully learned, treating compassion fatigue is a battle to be fought on many fronts. Mostly, it is a team effort, one that needs to be done with planning, compassion, and concerted effort. Remember that each person on your team could, at some point, be in need of the team's help as some degree of compassion fatigue is common to almost everyone in the helping professions. At the same time, it is up to you, the individual, to take the steps necessary to seek help *and* help yourself heal and move forward. No one can take your leap of faith for you; no one can embrace change for you; you must do it yourself.

CHAPTER 9:
BARRIERS TO TREATMENT

In spite of love, in spite of compassion, in spite of empathy, there is a cost for caring, and self-care covers the cost.

—Author Unknown

Treating compassion fatigue is not always easy or clear cut. Not surprisingly, many people who are told that they have compassion fatigue or discover the fact themselves are not open to treatment. Resistance to treatment is one of several barriers to treating compassion fatigue. This chapter will talk about these barriers to treatment, whether these barriers exist in a fellow employee, yourself, or within the very system where you work.

RESISTANCE FROM THE EMPLOYEE OR YOURSELF

Many a helpful HR department or supervisor has advised a worker to submit to an employee assistance program (EAP) or, outside professional help, only to encounter resistance from that employee. This resistance can manifest in the following ways: denial of the problem, anger, refusal to seek help, or discouragement.

In the same way employees ignore symptoms and resist treatment of compassion fatigue, you too can encounter this problem. In fact, a diagnosis of compassion fatigue in one's own self can be the most difficult to accept. While some of the symptoms we've already discussed are easy to recognize in others, when they happen in ourselves, they can be harder see and even harder to accept treatment for.

Here are a few reasons that helping professionals resist being treated for compassion fatigue:

- Lack of knowledge and understanding about compassion fatigue and your vulnerability to it
- Belief that you are somehow immune to compassion fatigue
- Belief (usually from your upbringing) that taking care of yourself is selfish
- Mistaken assumption that your physical and emotional symptoms are just personal shortcomings, that you may not be fit for this line of work
- Fear that opening up about your fatigue will cause a flood of distressful emotions
- Assumption that you alone are experiencing these challenges
- Fear that you will be identified as less than fit for service
- Shame about asking for help
- Conditioning that has told you not to ask for help
- Misconceptions about receiving professional help
- Past negative experience with a Therapist (EAP) with no background in Compassion Fatigue.
- Worry that your disclosures will not be held in confidence
- Fear of management reprisal because you disclosed problems

Love does not make us immune...

During most of my career, I operated under the notion that because I served out of love and compassion, I would be just fine. I believe helping others is God's work, and because I was doing God's work, nothing could happen to me. Or so I thought. In doing so, I overlooked counsel from men and women who were wiser than I, as well as from God's own teachings about rest and replenishment. I ignored my daily need to rest, refresh, and step away from helping others in order to quiet my mind, heal my body, and rejuvenate my spirit. I had been advised to care for my own temple so that I could continue to serve with peace, joy, and inner calm, but it was a command I mostly failed to heed.

My mission now: to educate about self-care

My mission now is to share what my life was like before and after I learned to take care of myself, to warn others of the potential dangers and to help them see alternatives to the way that too many helpers live and work. It is now my role to let others know that they can and should employ intentional self-care and self-regulation strategies. As helpers, we must make our wellbeing a priority so that we can remain vital and available to help those in need. You can, and should, use both planned and stolen moments during your day to calm and recharge your mind, body, and spirit.

Sometimes there is no real answer

Practicing adequate self-care seems so basic, yet so many of us fall short regarding our own wellbeing. Why? What are the barriers and blind spots preventing us from practicing adequate self-care? I have many of the possible reasons above (shame about asking for help, fear of management reprisal, etc.), and they help us identify why many resist being treated for compassion fatigue, but perhaps there is no real answer why so many of us fail to practice adequate self-care.

No excuses

Let me just say that as long as you work as a service provider and caregiver and are dealing with others' problems and traumas, until you address your own self-care, traumatic stress will forever manage you. Again, I plead with you to make a change now, if you aren't taking time out to care for your own wellbeing. Do it today. Really, that's as simple and direct as I can be, and practicing self-care is as simple as deciding to do it. So quit waiting and start caring for yourself. I know from personal experience that your life, both personal and professional, will improve once you do. Just do it!

SYSTEMIC BARRIERS

So, even if you are open to helping treat compassion fatigue in yourself or others who are close to you, you can still encounter barriers within your organization. And sometimes systemic barriers to progress can be the most difficult to manage because you are no longer dealing with a person but instead are dealing with an organization or a system.

Here are a few of the more common causes of systemic barriers to treating compassion fatigue:

- Absence of knowledge about compassion fatigue
- Organizational mission (or its absence) conflicts with coping strategies necessary for healing
- Denial that the condition even exists
- Expectation that staff can fix themselves in the face of overwhelming workplace demands
- Staff shortages and burgeoning worker caseloads
- Misplaced departmental priorities, where there is more concern about funding than treating impacted workers

- Little or no mechanism for staff to be able to process crises and tragedies
- Inadequate supervision to guide and support staff through work challenges
- Inconsistent organizational messages about self-care in the workplace
- Workplace culture that encourages workers to show no weakness and handle problems by themselves
- General resistance to any kind of change to the normal routine within the department
- Despite the realization of a departmental problem, a denial of its potential severity
- Inability to acknowledge the depth, reach, and detrimental implications of the problem
- Failure to recognize that well-supported staff equals a highly productive organization

As with the list for personal barriers to compassion fatigue, this list is far from exhaustive, but I think you may already recognize some of the above reasons if you have encountered resistance within your own department or organization.

COMBATTING SYSTEMIC BARRIERS

As I have mentioned before, not everyone everywhere is aware that compassion fatigue exists and that it can happen within their department or program, so departmental ignorance of compassion fatigue is real but can hopefully be remedied by education. Other reasons for systemic resistance can be a little trickier to resolve.

Strategies for combatting departmental resistance to treatment

The following are some strategies that organizations can use to combat departmental resistance to treating compassion fatigue. Please consider any or all that may apply to your organization:

Generalized training. Train all agency staff, including middle and senior management, about compassion fatigue: risks; recognizing the symptoms and early indicators in staff. Develop a trauma-informed work environment that supports prevention and treatment for recovery soon after traumatic experiences.

Specialized training. Conduct specialized training, one-to-one coaching, and support for supervisors so that they are well informed, skilled, and fully embrace their role to guide and support staff on the front lines of this very challenging and often disturbing and dangerous work.

Relationship awareness. Workers and supervisors need to understand their relationship, and supervisors must foster the professional growth and development of staff so that they remain qualified, effective, and highly motivated.

Staff orientation. New staff need to be thoroughly trained about compassion fatigue so that they will feel no stigma about the struggles they will inevitably experience on the job and to normalize the feelings that may arise as they encounter major crises. Most importantly, new staff should be encouraged to feel safe and confident that support is fully available to help them process, adjust, and move forward as they serve those in need.

Flexibility. Management should consider making staff roles flexible especially when some staff are being slammed with repeated horrific stressors. Permanent or even temporary shifts in assignments can help worker decompress and regulate emotionally and internally.

Team building. Organizations need to practice leadership team building across and up and down all hierarchical lines. Supervisors should be trained that all traumatic material, whether experienced by themselves or their subordinates, must be processed and released as part of recovery and resilience.

Continuing education. Ongoing staff training and development can reinforce the skills needed to cope with trauma as well as teach new skills and help prevent and heal trauma. The language and culture of the workplace should make clear that stressors are legitimate and that major concerns are part of the job, not the shortcoming of the individual.

Staff Retreats. Staff retreats should include strategies for release, refuel, review and recharge. In addition to fun morale-boosting activities, retreats should include refresher education about how the brain and body chemistry react to the stress hormone as well as body techniques and strategies for regaining self-regulation in the face of intensely stressful work experiences. Of course, every retreat, whether it is once or twice a year, should always include appreciations to *all* organizational staff.

Systemic barriers: my own story

As I have mentioned before, after my first episode of heart failure, I was reassigned to do community social work, which enabled me to work a typical 40-hour work, versus the 60+ hours/week I had grown accustomed to. Formerly, I often worked a 12-hour day, which of course included evenings. Under this new schedule, I complied with my cardiac care routine, ate healthy meals on schedule, and got a decent night's sleep.

After a couple of years, however, the organization started taking on more children in crisis and out-of-home placement. This was accompanied by a crushing increase in court visits, home visits, and documentation, which added many more hours (much of it on the road) to the workday and evenings. The in-house social workers were overwhelmed and overburdened, and they felt unfairly treated. I was asked to come back in-house to relieve some of their workload. At the same time, I still had community (children and youth) responsibilities, which were also quite time-intensive.

In no time, I lost my rhythm for self-care: I left home too early, and came home too late and too tired to take my prescribed morning walks. I also ate poorly and on the run, slept too few hours, and worked late into the evening on massive reports because I was worried about the children on my caseload.

Our organization's middle management listened to staff concerns, but their bosses at headquarters continued to require increased caseload numbers and recording add-ons that forced us to work harder. We asked if some of the redundant documentation could be taken off our plates, but this didn't happen. Morale was shot, tempers were flaring, and the collegial atmosphere formerly present among staff was deteriorating. That translated into a loss of supportive communications among staff. It was tense and rather cliquish. That to me and others was very hurtful and alienating.

Nevertheless, all of us continued to work hard for the sake of the children and youth who needed us. The pressures kept building, when two children died. One from coronary disease and another in a drive by shooting; and the toll was very heavy on everyone.

This contributed to my second serious episode of heart failure, which happened on the road while driving to my job. That day I never made it to work but instead I spent the next three months in intensive cardiac care.

WHAT IS THE LESSON IN ALL THIS?

The lesson in this is the same as it always is and the one I've been stating throughout this book: changes need to be made and fully embraced on the personal, professional, and systemic level to prevent and treat compassion fatigue and to make sure it doesn't recur.

CHAPTER 10:
PREVENTION

By understanding . . . compassion fatigue [as] the natural, predictable, treatable and preventable consequences of [caregiving] we can keep caring professionals at work and satisfied with it.
—Dr. Charles Figley 1995

Ironically, as caregivers and service providers, it is our caring and empathic nature that makes us susceptible to compassion fatigue. Therefore, knowing that compassion fatigue is predictable, my goal is to help the helper prevent this syndrome by taking self-care measures to recover from the stressors they encounter in their work and sustain wellness. In this chapter, I hope to help you to prevent compassion fatigue by practicing restoration and resilience as you serve and care for those impacted by traumatic life experiences.

PAY ATTENTION TO FAMILY HEALTH HISTORY

In addition to the emotional and psychological baggage we each carry with us from our families and our childhood, we each carry different health baggage as well. In order to help prevent compassion fatigue, you need to be aware of your own built-in health risks that you may be carrying.

In my own family, my birth father and maternal grandfather both dropped dead suddenly due to heart attacks (or heart failure) that apparently came out of nowhere. Neither of them were drinkers or smokers and they both walked everywhere daily (they both lived in New York City, where everyone walks and car ownership is not usually necessary). I had quit smoking some twenty years prior to my first heart failure. But at that time, I drank socially, walked infrequently (I drove everywhere), and I had a very stressful sit down job. To top it off, I also had the nerve to be significantly over weight. I did not consider myself a high risk cardiac candidate, even though I should have. And I did not consider my family history until after my own collapse and this wakeup call hit me with a wallop. So you can imagine going through this experience, I could not help but think that my time on earth was very possibly coming to a quick and painful end.

What not to do

Before my second heart failure, a colleague did a time study on the hours I devoted each week in committed activities. He carefully reviewed my hours on the job, the hours dedicated to my role as Christian education coordinator at my church and my social and family obligations, and he determined that I worked two and a half jobs during an average week. The graph he produced showed a 100 hour work week of committed waking activities. That meant that I slept an average of four hours per night when you factor in the nights that I actually had a restful and restorative sleep. I had been keeping this schedule for nine years. He warned me to stop. I was stunned and concerned but could no more stop than an alcoholic in denial. After my first collapse, I underwent a sleep study at the same medical center, which showed I was clearly operating under a dangerous level sleep deprivation and yet I persisted in serving with an unshakable, and unwise, determination.

Prevention requires paying attention to our bodies

Over the years I would have brief periods of sanity or rest breaks, which usually happened after I was physically drained and could do no more. I was blessed to have an insightful supervisor early in my child welfare career who allowed me to take administrative leave a couple of times a year, which would allow me to just stay home and catch up on some of the mountains off paperwork and avoid the phone calls that all demanded I resolve some crisis. When he departed for a career change, the twice-yearly habit that helped sustained me was over, and it was a downhill slide for me from that point on.

The only other times I slowed down were when I got sick. Physical ailments like an impacted wisdom tooth, the flu, or bronchitis with high fever were events that I could not push through, so I ended up staying home. These illnesses and health challenges appeared more frequently towards the end of my career and were a prelude to the first cardiac episode. I increasingly suffered from bouts of exhaustion, with me just falling asleep any time of day while sitting or even standing, sometimes as soon as it was time to drive to work first thing in the morning after my standard fair night's sleep. My body felt like I was carrying heavy sacks of rocks uphill. I was always breathless, had foggy states, and I had a relentless cough that alarmed everyone in my presence that I was possibly going to stop breathing at any minute. In retrospect, my body was screaming warnings to me. The signs were there and the red flags, if you will, were waving furiously, but I would not or could not heed the warning signs. I kept going, motivated by the needs of others and driven perhaps even more so by the serious degree of a crisis someone was facing.

Because I was faced with a near fatal illness, I had to stop living and working as I did and make a change. And the more self-reflection I give to this matter, the more it seems that the last time I had paid attention to my inner body was when I was carrying my children, some 30 years before. During my pregnancies, I wanted my inner womb environment to be safe and healthy and very calm for them. Now I must do the same just for me. So, with the help of close friends and advisors, I began to look at a variety of ways to do self-care. Now I have no more wiggle room or the "no time" excuses to continuing doing life as usual. I must conduct my life very differently. This I really want to do because I really want to live. I made a personal commitment and changed my life.

DOWNSIZING YOUR LIFE

Basically, to prevent compassion fatigue, or even to help treat it if you're already struggling with it, you should downsize your life. Here are a few things I did:

1. **Get rid of extra outside obligations.** I met with my pastor and with his blessing and support, I recruited, prepared, and passed the mantle of my role as Christian education coordinator at my church. This alone gave me back seven hours a week.

2. **Downshift at work if possible.** My employer restructured my job so that I could down shift at work. They hired another social worker to take over most of my foster children and family caseload, and I got more involved with the in-office training program as curriculum developer and instructor. This was stimulating and gratifying work, and most of all, it was healthier for me. Eventually, I soon transferred to community services for the same agency. In this new area,

the intense crisis-driven direct care responsibilities that exposed me to secondary traumatic events were limited. It is in this role that I benefited the most in terms of the reduced cardiac risk factors because I now worked normal hours. Primarily, I was able to work an eight or nine hour day. My case or agency involvement did not consume my thoughts day and night. I was better able to physically, mentally, and emotionally stop business at the end of the work day and simply be me, enjoying some normalcy and regulation in my life. Over time, these changes facilitated life patterns and structures that created what I surely felt as critical steps to recovery from heart failure.

3. **Take life slower.** I no longer rushed to work before dawn to tackle paperwork before the urgent calls started coming in. Instead, I rose in the morning and took a walk before my day started. It was amazing how much this grounded me and helped me organize my thoughts and make an action plan for the day. More importantly, it gave me greater sustained energy levels throughout the day and helped me sleep more soundly at night.

4. **Eat a healthy diet and regular meals.** I now eat three meals a day at normal hours. I had a good breakfast, often with the sun shining through my own kitchen window. This was a wonderful new experience for me to sit and eat quietly and slowly while gazing out the window at my garden and watching a humming bird or some other beautiful winged creature that visited me almost daily. I also ate lunch on schedule at work and was home most evenings at a respectable hour for dinner at my table. No more coming in at ten or later and eating something I barely had energy to throw together and then falling asleep sitting in the chair so that I did not risk suffocating myself by lying down and have food

back up into my windpipe. I marveled at how much I had missed so many years by not having this experience. I really treasured my peaceful and ordered mornings. Never again (I said) would I eat on the run by grabbing some honey coated cashews and diet caffeine soda from a gas station on the way to a home visit or emergency 30 to 100 miles away.

5. **Schedule in personal fun time and downtime.** I created a routine which included downtime with a book or a movie or simply quiet time. This downtime became a treasured time, and to my surprise it did not rob time from key responsibilities. I increased my hours of sleep. Now here is the real miracle: I began to have a life, sharing fun time with friends and taking quiet walks through the botanical gardens. I even discovered areas of my home, other than the kitchen, bathroom and bedroom, and I enjoyed living in these spaces. I am now balanced and am enjoying a healthy lifestyle.

Developing accountability partners

I mentioned having accountability partners in the chapter on treatment, but you need accountability partners for prevention as well, because if you want to maintain a healthy lifestyle, you will need additional people to help you. As I said earlier, your accountability partners should be picked from people who truly understand you and who will not allow you to isolate yourself or withdraw. Accountability partners should not need us to be the strong helper in their lives; rather, they should be mutually supportive friends. Accountability partners should themselves be living in a peaceful, joyful and refreshing space, so that they can periodically pull us back into a healthy space where you and they can mutually enjoy life. We need people who have the type of spirit that will help us rise to the surface and deeply exhale the distress and breathe in much laughter.

Of course, you will continue to care for your clients and loved ones as you can, albeit in a more balanced and mindful manner. However, while you are caring for others, make sure somebody is caring for you.

Intervention: The Continuum for Self-Regulation

As we stated earlier, learning to identify stress within your body and then performing a technique to reduce the stress, allows you to take care of yourself when others are not around to help.

Two important terms will help you see the imbalance associated with stress:

Regulation: this is the ability to experience and maintain stress within one's window of tolerance. This is generally referred to as being calm, regulated, or relaxed. This term is utilized by most scientific disciplines.

Dysregulation: this is the experience of stress outside of one's window of tolerance. Generally, this is referred to as being stressed out or in a state of acute or chronic distress.

It is good practice to learn to become aware of yourself and your stress level so that you can gauge which of these two states you are in at any time during your service and caregiving.

Dysregulation

Please understand that there are degrees of dysregulation: mild, moderate, and severe. Mild to moderate states of dysregulation can happen when you're late for work, stuck in traffic, or waiting in a long line at the DMV. When you're in a healthy state, you will realize that this unfortunate situation is temporary and resolvable, at which point, you have a good chance of calming yourself (self-regulating). In more severe states of dysregulation, you cannot see or realize an end to the distress. You will not be able to self-regulate without some form of intervention. By becoming aware of where you are on the spectrum, you can make healthier decisions about when it is time to step back, re-think possibilities, and rest your mind and body and refresh your spirit.

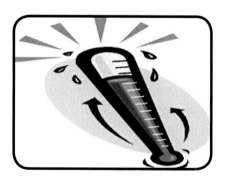

The dysregulated state can be experienced both in acute phases of stress and/or chronic phases of stress, and it is believed that "affect dysregulation" is a fundamental mechanism in all psychiatric disorders (Taylor 1998).

A single distressing event can bring on an acute state requiring one or more therapeutic interventions to help restore a sense of safety and inner calm and the capacity to move forward.

Chronic, or repetitive, phases of dysregulation require immediate therapeutic attention so that we can avoid prolonged states that often lead to more serious health concerns.

Self-Regulation

As my own case makes apparent, self-regulation is needed to help recover from and prevent compassion fatigue. And self-regulation is basically learning how to pay attention to stress cues within your body as well as stress triggers in your environment. Stress cues within your body include thought patterns, emotions, behaviors, as well as spiritual, interpersonal and physical cues. Stress triggers in your environment can come from your workspace, who you are meeting with that day, expectations by others, etc. After you consider both internal and external cues and forces, you then need to make adjustments so that you can return to a state of regulated emotional balance. In other words, you are gauging where you are at any given moment or situation.

To help you make adjustments and self-regulate, you should first gather baseline information about your regulated and dysregulated states. So, note and try to remember how you feel the next time you are going to begin a non-stressful appointment with someone, and then do the same the next time you are going to be in an intense or stressful appointment with someone on your caseload. Compare, if you can, how "regulated" you feel in both opposite situations. And then rate each on a scale of 1 to ten with 10 being the most intense level of stress and 1 being the least.

Doing a comparison will help you remember what it feels like to be regulated and what it feels like to go beyond your tolerance level. By being aware of your baseline, any shifts from regulated to dysregulated, and the level of dysregulation you are experiencing, you are now better able to regain a regulated state. In this way, you are now beginning to master your own self-regulation.

CHAPTER 11:
BLUEPRINT FOR SELF-CARE

Providing services to deeply troubled people is mentally and emotionally taxing and can wear our bodies out.

(Perry, 1998)

By now, you know that through diligently taking preventive measures we can better recover from the highly intense moments we encounter in our caregiving. But many times I hear from service providers that the short supply of time, money, and private space prevents them from practicing self-care. As a result of these concerns, I have taken the practices that my colleagues and I use to stave off compassion fatigue and have put together a blueprint that I use for proper self-care.

Here is a seven-point blueprint for self-care, whose steps you can follow daily to help prevent compassion fatigue.

1. Prepare: meditation and intention

Each day you need to get a good, restorative night's sleep. And then, before your workday starts, prepare yourself with a brief period of meditation. At first, five to ten minutes will do (20 minutes will come with practice). During this time, quiet your mind and still your body with three or more slow deep breaths. At this time, you will also want to set an intention for the day to accomplish two to three top priorities. Your health maintenance must always be one of your intentions. Write these down.

Make a written note of all tasks to be accomplished and be sure to check off what is completed. The brain loves to see checkmarks.

Remind yourself daily of the connectedness of the mind, body, and spirit and that you must give attention to the total you.

Suggestions for preparing

I. Settle down and quiet your home at least an hour before bedtime. Shut off toxic TV (e.g., the nightly news). If you (like me) sometimes need the television on to block negative images and thoughts so you can go to sleep, I recommend turning on some uplifting or humorous programming. Or, you can play some instrumental music to relax you. Make a written list of any unfinished business on your to-do list. By taking these concerns and putting them on paper your mind is better able to calm into a restful state known as Rapid Eye Movement (REM) sleep. Incorporate some aroma therapy with essential oils in a diffuser to fragrantly sooth your room, or rub a drop in the palm of your hands and hold them over your nose and breathe deeply as a last step when you lay down to sleep.

II. Use an area of your backyard or sit at your window in an area that is peaceful and pleasant to the eye. Early mornings, when the air is still relatively clear of automobile omissions is a good time. Take some cleansing breaths and just sit quietly with a positive quote, a scripture or an affirmation to meditate on. Keep your thoughts in the present, not only what the day holds for you.

III. First thing in the morning, dress for work then drive to your neighborhood park and take a short walk while meditating. Change from walking shoes to your work shoes when you return to your car. Do not walk fast enough to exert yourself and perspire. You simply wish to get some healthy blood circulation, cleansing breaths and a calming of your nervous system. This can also be done during the day at breaks and at lunch time.

IV. When the weather does not permit walking, sit in your car during a break or during lunch. Lower the window for fresh air and enjoy the quiet and "escape time" from work.

V. Sit up in bed the first thing in the morning and declare that this is your time. Have an affirmation or a scriptural book and a notepad and pen on the bed stand. Also have a CD with an inspirational message or calming music ready for playing. Begin your day with thanksgiving for the things you are happy about and grateful for. Read one of your chosen passages or listen to a brief recording. Close your eyes and take some deep breaths and think on these messages. Embrace them. Soak them in. After about ten minutes, some ideas for the day will float into your mind. This experience is somewhat like receiving a download. You will know these are things you wish to do so write them down.

When I prepare myself for each day, from the comfort of a prayer and meditation space I created in my guest bedroom, (before I had the guest room space to use, I did this from the comfort of a reclining reading chair I have in my bedroom), these so called downloads may from time to time become my intentions with the day. The amazing thing about this practice is that it helps me focus on the really important things. This practice also clears my mind to remember things that have slipped my mind. This can be very beneficial for those of you who like me are always multitasking.

No matter what tasks are facing you each day, work not to anticipate the worst case scenarios, but rather repeat to yourself, "I will do my best" and "I will be fine today." It is important to try and stay in the present and not focus on future events, which can overwhelm you. Follow the same thought processes for each of the suggestions for meditation.

Take a few minutes right now to identify and construct a personal plan for creating a sanctuary space for your meditation time. Be thoughtful about what *you* want that will bring you some peace and joy to your day, each day.

2. Impact control: check-ins

As we mentioned before, prior to, during, and after even the seemingly least stressful situations, you should always remain aware of your state of being so that you are consciously taking care of yourself, concurrent with the care you are giving to others. Even if traumatic stress occurs, you are now in position to manage and minimize the impact on yourself.

Suggestions for controlling the impact

I. Take a moment before any intervention such as a client/patient contact, a site visit, a meeting, or phone communication and check in with yourself. Even when the phone rings in your office and the ID window shows you the name of a particularly challenging personality on the other line, take a moment prior to answering (you can always call back immediately) to prepare yourself. Ask yourself "where am I in the moment?" "Am I okay?" "Am I ready for this?" Take some slow deep breaths along with your self inventory. Take a moment to depersonalize the behavior you may anticipate experiencing.

II. Remember that the grief, fear, and stress that drive the other person's undesirable behaviors is not really about you. It is not personal. Granted, their intention may be to make it a personal attack against you. However, you can decide not to accept this invitation. Remember to check your personal boundaries here too. Respectfully, and with kindness decide how people get to treat you.

III. Next, speak to yourself with positive affirmations: "I'm okay," "I'm doing well," "I've got this," and breathe while doing so.

IV. Check in with someone else: talk about your work with someone who cares about you and understands the nature of your work. This can be done without violating confidentialities. Talk about the situation and its impact on you without divulging the who, where, and when. Discussing your activities, your feelings, your frustrations and your successes can help you discharge negative emotions while allowing someone who cares about you to provide insight and support.

3. Bounce back

Bounce back speaks to the process of accelerated recovery, given that there is relatively little time to move from one demanding situation to the next. So I suggest some measures, many which involve a shift in thought process and an increase in positive internal dialogue that may help you get back to work quickly.

Two things need to happen in order for us to move forward quickly: first, we need to process or talk it out with peers, and second, we need to become aware of the physical impact of the external stressor we have just experienced.

Begin by doing a self-check along with proper breathing directed at the area(s) of your body where you are experiencing discomfort.

Suggestions for bouncing back

- If possible, spend some time using the tools of narrative and journaling to gain a deeper understanding of yourself. Look at how you just responded: physically, emotionally, cognitively, spiritually, and behaviorally, to the situation that just occurred. Through this process you not only learn to control the current stressor but also prepare yourself for future stressors.
- You will no longer repress the negative content and allow it to remain buried or stored inside of you while you pile on more and more distressing material over the course of the day(s). Instead, you will learn and grow and use the information in more productive new ways.
- Talk to a coworker or supervisor right away. De-compress by sharing your experience in getting immediate emotional support:
- Remember the chaos is theirs and not yours
- Remember the pain is theirs and not yours
- Remember to take responsibility for the delivery of quality service, not just the outcome

- Remember to use reasonable expectations and fairness to how you measure on-the-job success
- Remember to appreciate small successes
- Remember you are as important as the service you are giving
- Breathe while remembering and visualizing a beautiful place or scene
- Breathe while remembering an act of kindness towards you
- Breathe while thinking of someone you currently and actively love

4. Just say "No"

For many of us, no is the hardest word to say. As I have mentioned before about my personal history, many of us were wired to over extend ourselves and meet the needs of others before ourselves when we really should stop and rest. My parents and grandparents' self-sacrificing work and service ethic became mine.

Although life was very challenging during those times, it was much less complex than today and people weren't able to access us like they can today. Nowadays, extra demands on our time are far more pervasive and intrusive. Time for ourselves is all too limited. Therefore, we must be tenacious to carve out time and preserve it for ourselves.

Saying no and taking time for ourselves will allow us to be more present and effective. This will greatly increase our personal well-being and improve our delivery of service and caregiving to those in need.

Suggestions for saying "No"

- **Learn to say "No!"** Schedule down time for yourself throughout the day *and* sometime completely off during the weekend. Plan hard not to fill your weekend with a long list of tiring activities and tasks. Do this is in addition to the time you give yourselves to decompress after dealing with stressful clients or situations.
- **Guard your time**: make it a habit to be tenacious regarding *your* time. When you are at home, use your phone's caller ID and don't answer every phone call unless you know without a doubt that you must. Use judgment about which matters can wait, and which cannot. People who you think will be disappointed or resentful because you said 'no' or 'not now' to will get over it.
- Think about a time, person, or situation you have a hard time saying "no" to, and then write it down.
- List three reasons why you find it difficult to say "no."
- Would your saying no result in the loss of life, home, or health? If not, give yourself permission to say "no."
- Write down what it would take for you to say "no" when you need to take some out time for yourself.
- Share these reasons with your accountability partners. Allow them to talk about the benefits to you and help you through the ambivalence you feel about saying "no." Allow them to encourage your growth as a person who values your own self-care and well-being.

5. Evaluate: deep breathing

A few minutes of deep breathing will restore your body's homeostasis and bring you back to some normalcy after you have experienced stress. This is essential to your overall health and wellness. Because breath is the window to the nervous system, Dr. Anna Baranowski teaches a deep and slow breathing technique that is proven to be highly beneficial. Inhale deeply through the nose to the count of three, and then exhale completely through your mouth to the count of six. Please note that we each have different lung capacities, so the 3-6 breathing pattern may be a bit long for some. If that's the case, modify your breathing pattern to a 3-5 count or thereabouts. This method will relax your muscle tensions, regulate your respiration, lower your blood pressure, help you manage your emotions, and create inner peace both mentally and physically.

Suggestions for evaluating

You may have noticed that your body tenses up (or constricts) during stressful events. This restricts blood flow, can cause abdominal discomfort, or headaches, etc. and makes it difficult to focus. A beneficial skill (Jacobson, 1934) is to use a tense to relax process. Follow these guidelines to perform this process:

I. Take two slow deep breaths.

II. On the third inhalation tighten (clench) your right arm from the shoulder to your hand and hold tightly for two to three seconds. As you exhale, relax fully and let your arm drop. Repeat these four steps with your left arm, your right then left leg, and then your entire body. In seconds you will relax your body and clear your mind.

III. Put web alerts to pop up on your computer/lap top at intervals throughout the work day, and at home that will cue you to take some deep and slow calming breaths.

IV. Have your workplace accountability partners cue you to breathe and/or tense to relax periodically throughout the day.

V. Scan your body from head to foot for tightness or aches, and discomforts after a stressor. This is practicing body awareness of where stress attacks your body.

VI. Whenever you experience a disquieting sensation often accompanied by an emotion, place your hand over that area, focus your thoughts on it and breathe into that area. This method will help you clear your body and mind of toxic blocks or buildup.

6. Recharge

Once you have completed the stressful interaction and have returned yourself to a state of calm, it is time to recharge and build up positive and joyful experiences that will continue to provide a foundation of wellness. You should continuously recharge your energies when working in a challenging profession or caregiving for loved ones so that you have a core of optimism and resilience to get you through difficult times. The following are a few suggestions to help you recharge:

- **Comedy and fun**: participate in activities that are filled with humor and fun, like comedy movies or books, comedy clubs, crazy joke-a-minute friends, table games, music, and dancing.
- **Hobbies**: take part in hobbies and special interests that capture your attention and distract you from thoughts about work and service. These could be arts and crafts, hiking, sightseeing, rock climbing, dancing, gardening, sports watching or activities, etc. Visiting botanical gardens and museums are both favorites of mine. These activities can recharge your battery while providing intellectual and recreational stimulation.
- **Speak words of thanksgiving**: caregiving often demands that you mentally replay unfortunate incidents as you keep

appointments and prepare case reviews, written reports, and case recordings, etc. Combat this by frequently speaking words of thanksgiving aloud and in your mind. Give thanks for what did not happen in the same situation, or give thanks for positive aspects of your life. Shifting your internal dialogue to the positives becomes something of a protective factor for you when future stressors appear.

- **Give and receive affection**: Giving and receiving affection can also recharge your spirit, body, and mind. Because the skin is the largest and heaviest organ of your body, and all sensory pathways lead to its surface, touching or hugging another human being or a loving pet is magnificently calming. Giving and receiving affection positively changes brain chemistry, much like installing a new battery in a clock that has stopped.

7. Appreciate: passion for life

Appreciating life and getting involved in the activities that provide you with passion and excitement can help restore you and are necessary for inner strength and readiness. You can easily reignite your passion for life by appreciating beauty. The key is to do it now: don't wait until you feel like it; do it until you feel like it. Here are a few suggestions to do this:

- **Create art**: you can create beautiful things even if you think you have limited talent. This can be anything, from working with paints, clay, needlepoint, knitting, woodworking, etc. The brain chemicals released during the creative thinking process are healing balm for your spirit mind and body.
- **Go sightseeing**: visit or use media to gaze on panoramic scenery such as waterfalls, mountains, the sky and seascapes.
- **Indulge in music**: indulge in music that delights your spirit.

STRATEGIES FOR SELF-CARE AT WORK

You can practice self-care at work, especially when you encounter clients or patients with issues that act as triggers for you. This process includes some advance preparation but will prepare you and hold you accountable for your own self-care. By taking these steps, you acknowledge the process and gain control of the impacts on yourself.

Remember, that as the professional in charge, you can terminate an interview or temporarily suspend an interview if you feel heightened tension that makes it difficult to continue. But if the stress is obvious but not debilitating, here are a few things you can do to lower your stress level while staying engaged with your client.

Strategize and develop a template

- **Plan**: plan a structure for the interview with areas you need to discuss, questions you want to ask, and specific behaviors, tasks, and updates that you want to focus on.
- **Focus**: find a focal point such as a picture on the wall, your notepad, or an object of interest on your desk that you can glance at intermittently to remind you to self-calm.
- **Use props**: get props ready that you can use to help you relax when you are with the client. These could be a glass of water or a stone to manipulate in the palm of your hand. If there is carpet under your desk, step out of your shoes and gently massage your feet into the texture, or use a pen to take notes or doodle during the interview.
- **List in-between tasks**: make a list of things you will do between the stressful interview and your next appointment. You can take a brief walk, listen to music, meditate, process with someone, or do some 3-6 breathing, etc.

- **List end of the day activities**: list activities you will do at the end of the day to relax and decompress. All of the activities listed in the previous section on self-care are appropriate here (meditation, recharging, mind/body work, etc.)
- **List weekly and monthly activities**: list things you will do weekly, monthly, and bi-monthly that restore and revitalize you. These can be vacations, movies and theater, hikes, and crafts or (fun) educational projects.

SOME MORE TOOLS FOR RESTORATION

In addition to all the interventions I've given you, here are a number of additional seemingly small yet effective tools for you to use for recovery, prevention, and recharging.

Cognitive negative awareness: be aware of ruminating on negative thoughts. Block these with music, a bit of humor, or even a few minutes of positive conversation.

Relaxation: Step away from the desk or immediately after a client or patient interaction, breathe deeply, stretch, take a short walk, and quiet your mind (this takes practice). It is important not to carry the negative aspects of what you just left. Block the negative thoughts and replace them with more positive thinking, or simply hum a song. You should quiet your mind for five to ten minutes frequently during your day.

Mindfulness: before any interview or event, ask yourself "where am I in the moment?" and do what you need to do for *you first*. Being mindful of yourself will help you to respond mindfully to the needs of the people you serve.

Creating narratives: team up with coworkers and your supervisor to develop some scripted positive responses to negative client behaviors. Test these and always be willing to adjust them according to the client's responses or their ability to resonate with what you are saying. More verbally assaultive clients can cause you to struggle with an appropriate and effective response. This is one way to build a repertoire of responses that can counteract or replace difficult communications with better outcomes.

Exercise: We've seen excellent results when the practices of martial arts such as Tai Chi, Tae Kwon Do, Q-gong are used because these forms of exercise always foster proper breathing. In addition, walking, swimming, bike riding, and gym workouts are also very effective exercises.

Baroque classical music: the structures of these particular music chords and rhythms have a powerful effect on the body's capacity to regulate and de-stress.

Reading: after a highly stressful day, books, especially light or fun reading, have a glorious capacity to take you away on another life adventure.

Dance: is a therapy! The chemical release from the joy of dancing is highly beneficial

Feeding your spirit: immerse yourself in a love relationship with your creator, your source of spirituality. Caregiving is much easier and lighter with a personal spiritual foundation, especially when you consider the dark places we visit both physically and mentally and the painful measures we often times have to take.

Thera-play: play is highly therapeutic, so reconnect with toys and games that formerly gave you pleasure (yo-yo, swings, monopoly, train sets, doll or action figure collections, race cars, hula hoops, card games, silly putty, sandbox, etc., etc.)

Nutrition: eating can become a negative coping habit for many caregivers. Stress creates high acidity in our bodies, so consider eating more foods with high alkaline levels (cucumbers, avocados, lettuce, tomatoes, broccoli, onions, etc.,) to balance the acids. And, as often as you can, make food choices that nurture and heal your body rather than just temporarily soothing the stress.

Breathing: I want to direct you to a demonstration on the simple and seemingly automatic act of breathing. Paying attention to and manipulating the breathing process can help you with stress. Deep and well-paced breathing can help you create inner calm when faced with highly stressful situations. It is also an important technique to employ prior to facing a potentially difficult interaction and immediately after the interaction.

Using a method I'd like you to view, you can better control your state of mind. Please watch the video of Dr. Anna Baranowski and practice the technique along with her. You may be surprised at how effective this is. You can view this technique on YouTube. It is called "Breath Training: 3-6 Breathing: The Window into the Nervous System."

Release, recover, and recharge

Each of the aforementioned techniques and strategies I have provided could easily overlap or fit into any of the principal goals of good self-care. They are release, recover, and recharge. The following table contains a sample template for you to use in designing your own self-care template.

Release	Recover	Recharge
Process debrief	Restoration Refuel	Resilience
Talk it out	Breathe	Prayer Meditation
Cry, yell, holler	Narrative Telling the story	Play activities
Body check	Meditation	Humor
Journal	Humor	Creative arts
Breathe	Prayer	Dance music listening
Walk/gentle exercise	Modifying internal dialog	Socialize for pleasure

ANCHORING OUR UNDERSTANDING OF THE MIND AND BODY EFFECT

Hopefully, I am leaving you in a more relaxed state and most importantly with knowledge and skills that will help get you there any time you need to re-establish a sense of inner calm.

When action plans do not work or when resources are in short supply (or nonexistent), it is easy for us to feel very frustrated and that we are failing our clients. It is at these times that I've learned to practice what I call rethinking positive. I urge you to remind yourself that you are giving each of your clients or patients, even in these very difficult times, the experience of you. And that experience is very different from any they have ever had. They are in the presence of you and in receipt of your compassionate spirit.

I believe I can give small words and acts of kindness to someone who has experienced a trauma. These words and acts are a lifeline and allow me to plant a seed of resilience in each of my clients: the soft acceptance in my face and body posture, or just listening to them express their pain and acknowledging their hurt. I also acknowledge their courage in the face of so much pain, while offering to sit and be with them under the horrific weight of their pain.

For my part, I now acknowledge also my pain that I feel for them and for the horror of the experience they suffered. I now get to transform my feelings. I get to rewrite the story and the ending. For instance, when someone was physically or sexually brutalized I tell myself that their mind (as an act of protection) went to a secret safe place where they were not present during the horror. In cases of kidnapping, violation, or torture of children, I tell myself that angels were present in that moment. I tell myself that the child victim was preoccupied and at peace in the presence of the angels, temporarily unaware of the horror happening in the natural world.

I still had to come to terms with the deaths in tragedies like 9/11 and do so in a way that would allow me to still be helpful, even though this one event became one of my breaking points. So many of the youth I counseled in groups after were deeply troubled by the people who were forced to leap to their deaths to escape the intense heat and flames. I said to myself that seconds after that leap those precious souls separated from their bodies and took flight into the arms of angels. I told myself that they never hit the bottom.

Similarly, the tragedies in Sandy Hook and every other school or shopping mall massacre struck pain in my heart. Now, I check very hard and don't allow my thoughts to constantly replay images and sounds of those children having been terrified and suffering while watching one another's demise. Instead, I choose to transform that story, and I say to myself and believe in my heart that they probably heard a very loud and shocking noise, but they didn't know what happened. And before they could realize what happened, their precious souls took flight in the arms of angels.

I use my thought processes and my empathy to be in the space that allows me to have some personal resolution, and then as quickly as possible, I shift my love back to those who are left behind and need my help to cope with unimaginable loss.

PREVENTION MUST BE LIFELONG

As I have said before, prior to my first cardiac failure, I was a social worker with a caseload and responsibilities for other adjunct agency services. These responsibilities included cross-cultural specialist, curriculum developer, and educator to foster children. It was this last role, educator to foster children, which taxed me the most. My main job was to help these children compete academically, but I quickly became aware that most of these children had their self-worth broken by routine abandonment and their normal assumptions of safety shattered through unspeakable violations to their innocence.

With this unsettling knowledge I worked hard to make a difference: the hours, the efforts, the heartbreaks, the successes, the short-lived pieces of progress, and the accomplishments were all par for the course. But my failure to count the cost of this work on my health and well being and my failure to attend to my own self-care resulted in my nearly fatal health collapse.

Upon my return to work, my managers, out of concern for my well-being and to keep me employed, changed my workload and gave me a new assignment. In my new assignment I was a community social worker, linking, collaborating, and coordinating education and health services for children in the foster care system. I had a relatively normal work schedule for two years and a better chance to add a stable routine and balance to my life that I had not experienced in years. I was now able to balance consistently my responsibilities and self-care habits. Of course, child welfare emergencies sometimes still interrupted my flow, requiring frequent adjustments in priorities. As you know now, with my propensity for self neglect, I easily put myself at the back of the line in my list of priorities. Additionally, I had this pointed out to me by my best sister friend: I had over identified with my role as helper, making this role my entire identity. My sister friend opened my eyes, letting me know that I am Beverly and that while I'm at work, I put on the role of social worker, and that I should take that role off when I'm not at work. This is easy to say, but not easy to do. But I was feeling better and the new work assignment and schedule had been working for me.

At the near end of two years, the direct foster care services clinical team began to feel overwhelmed with case responsibilities. Perhaps they were down in staff numbers, I can't remember, but the consensus was that because I had a clinical degree I should come back in and assume some of the case load. The management team, out of concern for my health, assured me that I would have the support I needed, and they did the best they could. But with the nature of child welfare work being what it is, and I being who I am, I fell quickly back into my former work patterns.

Neither I nor my team were aware that, once compromised, the muscles in and around my heart and lungs were now *more* vulnerable to stress. So it was a few months later, on the way to work one morning on the freeway, I felt my seat belt suddenly get very tight across my chest. I tugged on it a few times, hoping to lengthen it and relieve some of the pressure. I next noticed I was having difficulty inhaling, combined with sudden extreme exhaustion. I suddenly wanted to lay my head down on the steering column and sleep. I knew with horror that I had to get off the road or I was going to die at the wheel and possibly kill other drivers. This was difficult because I was in the middle lane, and the cars to my right were totally in rush hour mode.

I had to decide quickly before I passed out what to do. I carefully forced my way into the right lane, fully expecting a fender bender, and pulled off onto the side of the road. Happy that I had not killed anyone, I surrendered to the exhaustion. I thought I was dying, but some time later I woke up.

Now I'd really done it. Heart failure part two landed me in three months of intensive cardiac rehabilitation care. My protocol required me to visit the rehab center three times per week. At the rehab center, I endured workouts I thought would kill me where I experienced breathing difficulty and sensations of weakness to the point of passing out. At home, I lived in a recliner day and night just to be able to breathe.

I was so angry and disappointed with myself for once again coming to this near fatal state. I also was concerned because I was suffering with depression, likely resulting from my body's loss of capacity and the drastic changes this forced on my life. Yes, I spent some time in a pity party too. However, I was driven to find out why this again happened to me.

So, I began researching about stress, because I felt that knowing as much as I can about this condition would allow me to see risk factors and warning signs so I could predict and thus prevent another episode of heart failure. Again, because what is predictable is preventable, I want each of you to have the information to make healthy choices in your life. And the key to making healthier choices is knowing the dangers of unmanaged traumatic stress.

Today, I am so much better than my pre cardiac days. My heart failure and the fact that I lived to research, study, write training materials, and teach about compassion fatigue made an incredible difference in my wellbeing. I really enjoy the going to the movies and having the neighbors over Friday nights or Saturday evenings for videos and snacks or joining them for breakfast out on Saturday mornings. I love having idle time to think about what I whimsically want to do or not do. I had finally learned not to fill in a tight space in my calendar with unfinished work, a new request, or social obligations. I had learned to breathe and fully exhale.

CHAPTER 12: HEALTHY HABITS MOVING FORWARD

Rest and self-care are so important. When you take time to replenish your spirit, it allows you to serve others from the overflow. You cannot serve from an empty vessel.

–Eleanor Brown

Once you feel you are managing your compassion fatigue, it is time to think about maintaining healthy habits moving forward: right eating, sufficient sleep, exercise, play, and spirituality, just to name a few areas you need to care for.

RIGHT EATING

One of the foundations of good mental and physical health is eating right. The old saying 'you are what you eat' is still true. In general, avoid refined sugars, refined flours, artificial additives, and too much red meat or animal products. Books and books have been written on what we should and shouldn't eat, so opinions vary, but most Americans eat too much sugar, too much meat, too many white flour products (like bread), and not enough fresh fruits or vegetables.

Three simple techniques

If there are three simple techniques you can do right now that will improve your health without having to go on a fancy or restrictive diet: avoid eating fast food, drink more water, and avoid drinking soda.

Of these simple techniques, avoiding fast food should be obvious given what they tend to contain: sugars, artificial additives, saturated fats, refined flours, and processed animal products. The temptation to eat fast food is there because these foods are fast and easy and relatively cheap. But you should resist that temptation. Fast food is not your friend. A good way to avoid eating fast food is to prepare your own lunch, or at least to find alternatives at your work cafeteria, if you have one, or in the food vendors near where you work where the food is more natural. But the best bet is still to prepare your own food.

The need for water, however, might seem a little less obvious, but adequate hydration is essential to good health. Our bodies consist of between 50% and 75% water. Drinking water instead of coffee, soda, or sugar-laden fruit juices can also help you maintain your weight and help your body cleanse itself. One online study followed a woman who drank at least a half quart of water in the morning and evening. After one month of drinking more water she looked younger, felt healthier, and her digestion improved.

And last but not least, everyone should avoid drinking soda. Carbonated beverages often contain sugars, artificial flavors and colors, or artificial sweeteners and other chemicals designed to enhance flavor or experience. These beverages can also contain carbonic and phosphoric acids, which are not good for you. The sugars and the acids in soda drinks can erode your teeth and cause digestive issues. And the calories and sugars in sodas have been shown to cause weight gain and contribute to type 2 diabetes. If you do a quick online search, you will find overwhelming evidence against drinking soda along with dozens of ill effects that soda consumption can cause.

Again, eating right need not cost you a lot or be complicated. It can be as simple as reaching for a piece of fruit instead of a candy bar, or having a glass of water instead of a soda.

SUFFICIENT SLEEP

Multiple research studies have linked even short term sleep deprivation to increased risk for stroke, heart disease, obesity, cancer, accident proneness, mood swings, memory impairment, and loss of brain tissue. Regular good sleep habits each night is essential to health. Make list of unfinished business; the "to do list" before bed each night. By taking these concerns out of your head, and placing them on paper, your mind is better able to clear and calm for a good night's sleep. Warm fragrant foaming baths, soothing non-lyric music sounds and aroma therapy is also helpful for deep restorative sleep. While time frames vary with age, we should ideally have 3-5 periods of REM (Rapid Eye Movement) sleep each night; each lasting 1-2 hours per period. This is regenerative sleep.

EXERCISE

As with diet, books and books have been written on proper exercise. And as with diet, opinions vary as to the proper amount and the proper exercise. The most I want to say here is that your exercise needs to have two elements: it needs to be realistic, and you need to do it regularly. If you don't have time to exercise daily, you should exercise at least three times a week. I have friends and associates who do nothing more than take a vigorous walk for at least 30 minutes each day. If that is all you have the time, energy, or resources to do, you will improve your health. If there is a sport you like to play, if you enjoy working out, or if you have other aerobic exercises, like running, biking, or swimming that you can do, then do them. Be sure to choose exercise that is appropriate for you. You will know this when you experience greater energy levels, rather than fatigue, throughout the day. Again, the principle is to exercise regularly and do something that won't injure you or cause you to get discouraged and quit.

PLAY

Forget not that the earth delights to feel your bare feet and the winds long to play with your hair.

–Khalil Gibran

I have mentioned this earlier, but play is important. Play is what helps us stay human, and it's what we do to rejuvenate ourselves, recharge our batteries, and let our minds and bodies rest and recover. As a caregiver, you are faced with others' problems every day, and so regular play is essential for recharging your body, mind, and spirit.

What do I mean by play? Hobbies, games, and innocent diversions all count as play. As I have mentioned earlier, I enjoy dance and painting, and I get much revitalization from doing both.

What play isn't: play isn't just sitting down in front of the TV or consuming a large amount of alcohol. Healthy play also isn't participating in potentially damaging pursuits like gambling. Play should be fun, productive, healthy, and safe for it to benefit you. If it's been so long since you've played that you don't remember what you like to do, then take some time to rediscover yourself.

SPIRITUAL HABITS

Only from silence can come the depth of expression, the well-spring of beautiful and common language that will help us interpret all the sounds of the noisy world.

—Rev Daniel P. Coughlin,
(prayer at the opening session of Congress, April 23, 2009)

We've talked about physical and social habits, now let's talk a little about spiritual habits.

Feeding my spirit daily: Letting peace by my guide

After my second episode of heart failure, I developed a theory, which I nicknamed 'in spite of' (or ISO). 'In spite of' reminds me that I can only do so much when it comes to working within a system. It acknowledges politically and fiscally dismantled programs, drastically reduced resources, and caseload numbers that far exceed ideal case management.

Then I asked the Spirit of God to help me know see what I can do I can do in spite of what is not available from the system. My ISO theory says that when resources have dried significantly, my respect, kindness, support, and encouragement still go a long way. Many times I have been able to take pleasure knowing that I can give of myself: my caring; my listening, my understanding, my help, and my knowledge of available resources or alternatives for clients. This is possible for me when I know without a doubt that I have the grace and power from my source, a loving God who has equipped me to care deeply for the struggling and suffering in humanity. The most precious element in the cornerstone of my spiritual life is a spirit of gratitude for what God has given to me to give to others.

Mornings seem to work best

Personally, I start each day connecting with my source by praying and meditating in a quiet area of my home I designed just for me and the Spirit of God. My meditation space, which is a section of a rarely used guest room, is peaceful, serene, and decorated in such a way that I can transcend the hectic world and feeling wrapped in the grace of the holy Trinity, who knows my every need and who listens intently to me. In these moments I feel strengthened to face whatever the day holds. This also sets the tone for my entire day. I feel organized, clearer in my thinking, more confident in my capabilities, and able to face challenges and maintain an inner calm born of an assurance that I am not alone.

I do this every morning because I have not been successful protecting this time later in the day, as the many tasks and issues that arise during the day make it difficult for me to find time to slow down, completely quiet my mind, and meditate. My meditation works best for me at the start of my day. After I start my day this way, throughout the day I reflect on my source and whisper words acknowledging the presence and a word of thanksgiving.

So, I recommend mornings as the best time to feed your spirit, and I encourage you each to feed your spirit in your own special way.

SUMMING UP

As you can probably see, no doubt both from your own experiences as well from reading about mine, you need to be vigilant in your self-care after you recover from compassion fatigue. Had I heeded the advice in this chapter and lived more in accordance with the way mother nature intended us to live—right food, adequate sleep, exercise, play, and attention to my spirit—I might not have had my second relapse.

CHAPTER 13:
FAMILY CAREGIVERS

In dealing with those who are undergoing great suffering, if you feel "burnout" setting in, if you feel demoralized and exhausted, it is best, for the sake of everyone, to withdraw and restore yourself. The point is to have a long-term perspective.

–Dalai Lama

Much of the time, family caregivers get little or no support from other relatives due to distance, conflicting responsibilities, financial constraints, family conflicts, or simply an absence of compassion. Therefore, this chapter is for two groups. First, it is for those who are employed in the helping professions but who also act as family caregivers, which puts you at even greater risk of succumbing to compassion fatigue. Second, it is for those who act as family caregivers but have no professional training in the human services, for you face many of the same challenges, struggles, and risk factors of compassion fatigue as those in the helping professions. The self-care strategies skills and methods recommended throughout this chapter (and this book) still apply very much to you.

MY LONELY JOURNEY OF DETERMINED LOVE

The call came in the middle of the night. My youngest son Jamal, who was living in California, was brought into the hospital in a near fatal state. I left New York City and was in California by his side within 30 hours. As is the case with so many family caregivers, this would be an arduous journey that I would embark on mostly by myself. However, I must hasten to add that there were those who drove us daily for three months on a 5-hour round trip for specialized medical treatments. And there were also distant family and loving friends who diligently checked in on me and my son; their kindness and encouragement over a vast distance, coupled with my faith, sustained me. Truly, being a family caregiver can be a dramatic and stressful undertaking, and it can also be a life-altering undertaking.

I've often wondered why some members of a family constellation are identified by others in the family as "the one" who will take care of those most in need. In my case, perhaps it was because I was the oldest of three daughters that I had always assumed the caregiver role. And because of this, I was perceived as too strong to need any help or support. I remember, on the rare occasion that I would call another family member to talk about a deep concern I was facing, that I would be told—in jest almost—that I was the strong one and that I would get through it. End of story.

Just hours before I left for California to see Jamal, I called a relative to share that I would be away and my upset about his illness. After I had told them what was happening and paused briefly to catch my breath, my loved one said "let me tell you about my day." I was thunderstruck. It was obvious that they had not even listened or if they had, they may have been unable to comprehend that I was experiencing trouble. I did not think that this was insensitivity on their part; rather, I think that they perceived me as the strong one, the one who had no problems, the one who could fix or manage everything, so they could not grasp that I was in distress. They could only express their own distress and need for my support, which is what they had usually done when talking with me.

And of course, me being the helper that I am, I never wish to burden anyone with my problems, so I did not push the conversation to make them understand what was going on, that I was terrified for my son. Instead, I calmly and politely ended the conversation after listening to their concerns and made some helpful suggestions, and I kept my feelings to myself. This was one of my loneliest moments; however, I pushed it down so deeply that I did not think about it for several more months but let myself be caught up in the myriad of activities and decisions over the battle for my son's life. After the phone call was over, I quickly shifted my thoughts to getting to my son as quickly as I could to help him through what would be a two-year battle for his life.

I later became aware that no one (with one exception) else in that particular family network or surrounding area had ever called to ask about my son, or myself. I assumed no one knew what was happening to us, and for reasons I cannot explain, I did not make them aware. I was in no way angry; I just became insular about what needed to be done for my child while maintaining our financial stability. More than a decade later, I learned that some members of my family perceived my disappearance from New York to California to care for my son as abandonment.

Today, I ask myself how I let so much time go by disconnected from people I really love. While I do very much regret being unavailable for them, I also did not miss the fact that some of them were not available for me; I simply did not notice. Being a professional service provider working with others' trauma and tragedy while also being a family caregiver seemed to lock me in a time warp where I did not realize the loss of precious time and connection with my family.

Disconnecting from my family and friends

The risk of disconnecting from your family is high in service work. Few people outside our work, including our spouses, partners, and closest family members, understand the scope and gravity of tragedies that exist in our country or the daily numbers of injured parties that come to us for help. Nor do they wish to hear about the suffering and tragedy we face.

Over the years as I worked in my job, I became preoccupied by the stories, the scenarios, and the needs of my clients, and in so doing became disconnected from many of my own family. This happened, not usually because others did not want to hear, but because I chose not to talk about my work, and so I missed a chance to bounce back and recover by talking with them. At the end of most work days, I was mentally and emotionally consumed with work concerns; I would re-live therapy sessions, time spent negotiating with struggling clients reasoning with injured and angry parties, as well as time spent dealing with my coworkers and the challenging and ever-changing systems I worked under.

Because I had spent my day mentally and physically absorbed in helping to rescue, protect, and help the children, youth, and adults I served to heal, I had no conversation left in me when I got home. At times, I was unable to engage in even the simplest, casual conversations. I actually grew to hate the phone when I got home. Never did I just call up a friend to ask what was going on. Because my thoughts were overflowing with negative and distressful content along with my action plans to address this content , there was no space and certainly no energy for lightweight banter, and I didn't want to talk to anyone. I couldn't hold a phone to my ear for one more second.

Again, it was nothing personal against my family or friends. All I wanted was quiet. As a result of my work concerns, it was all I could do to generate the energy to meet my responsibilities to my children, spouse, and home. I did manage of course aided by love; however, there were many days and evenings when I functioned on auto-pilot. In the end, it was I who set the precedent for too little connection with friends and extended family.

THE PERSONAL, EMOTIONAL, AND PHYSICAL INVESTMENT OF FAMILY CAREGIVERS

In the USA alone, there are approximately 101.2 million family caregivers, of which 40 million are baby boomers. Many are not only just a paycheck away from potential financial ruin, but many also face challenges to their emotional and physical health, and statistically, many of them suffer declining health, which may surpass the health challenges of the loved ones they are caring for.

Caring for your aging mom and dad

Almost as bad as losing your parents to death, witnessing them losing their independence is often painful and distressing, especially when they lose their dignity or experience great suffering as their lives near their end.

Thus it should come as no surprise that caring for aging parents is fraught with difficulty and can become overwhelming if you are also juggling the demands of family and work. Sadly, your life and health needs often take a back seat to the chronic needs of your loved one. Add to that the guilt and societal expectation to care for the people who once cared for you, and it becomes hard to say "no" when asked to help your mommy and daddy.

Some of the responsibilities that those caring for aging parents include:

- Transporting them to appointments
- Medication management
- Oxygen machine supervision
- Personal care, wound care, and hygiene care
- Sitting at bedside during hospitalizations
- End of life care
- Navigating systems for services for the vulnerable
- Managing conflicting opinions and strife from other family members
- Financial planning, management, and support
- Providing a residence or homecare
- Providing or managing basic housekeeping
- Shopping
- Companionship
- Safety supervision (e.g., preventing them from wandering off or falling)

If you are caring for aging parents, know that your privacy, intimacy, and family plans are all subject to compromise. I have witnessed colleagues, friends, and my own family members undergo mood and personality changes while caring for aging parents. I have also witnessed their declining peace, joy, and health. And while a few have walked away from caring for their parents, most do not give up, sustained as they are by their own faith or determination not to give up. Yet all those who care for their parents, including those who eventually quit, find that their lives change dramatically, often in unexpected ways.

for those who continue caring for their parents, they must be careful to care for themselves. Many who press on through sheer determination often stop asking for help. And others, fed up with waiting for other family members to step up, often make the mistake of counting only on themselves to get things done. But instead of relying on themselves alone, they should mindfully decide to slow down and find ways to rely on others such as community resources to get much needed respite. When caring for aged parents, you must make it a habit of stepping backback and catch your breath, rest, and eventually recover so that you can attend to other pressing responsibilities.

The following website has many helpful suggestions for those who care for their parents:

http://www.aarp.org/supportcaregivers

Caring for sick children

When they are very young, our children are of course completely dependent on us. But when a child becomes very ill, being a parent becomes even more of a challenge. When a child is fighting for its life, the parents join and lead that fight as well. Whether the illness is cancer or some other life threatening or life-altering diseases, a mental or emotional illnesses, developmental challenges, and other special needs, caring parents can struggle on many fronts: from navigating medical and mental health systems and complying with frightening and painful treatment protocols, to managing home and work responsibilities and meeting the needs of other family members, the work of a parent with a sick or needy child is never done. And last but not least, as a parent with a sick and/or special needs child, you are also continually encouraging your child, even when fraught with uncertainty yourself, and assuring them that you will always be there for them.

Grandparents who care for children

Due to a family crisis, breakdown, or tragedy, some older citizens can find themselves raising their small grandchildren. This can be quite challenging for many reasons. At the outset, their grandchildren's grief and fear-driven behaviors are quite challenging for the grandparent(s). This is compounded by complex losses for all parties and the fatigue experienced from the constant demands that childcare produces. This situation is also the complete antithesis of how an aging retired adult expected to be spending their later years of life.

MY STORY

I remember well the day Jamal started crying incessantly. I knew that something was wrong with my seven-month-old baby, because he had always been a happy, playful, and contented baby. I checked him myself from head to toe to see what could be the matter, and then I quickly called his pediatrician. At first, she insisted that he was fine because babies cry. But I argued vehemently that his persistent crying was unusual and very different from crying due to gas or restlessness. He had no rash, no sores, and there was no accident or injury, and he refused to eat or drink.

My pediatrician, and a urologist who was called in on emergency, discovered that my baby was acutely suffering from a birth abnormality that had gone undetected. At this point, Jamal was in a near fatal state. The urology surgeon told me that my child's life was in peril, but he had an experimental procedure he had developed and wanted to try that *may* save his life. My decision required passionate prayer, a debate with my husband, and a consultation with my father, who was 3000 miles away, via phone. My decision to move forward also was aided by the sincere compassionate, concern, and determination in the eyes of the physician, one Dr. Richards P. Lyon.

My inner spirit said that this tall, kindhearted man, who is still a friend some 43 years later, was sent to us as the hands of God. Not only did he save my child's life, but he always inquired about my wellbeing and made accommodations for my comfort, especially during the many times that I flew with Jamal from New York City to California for one of his many surgeries.

Truly, my challenges and struggles as a parent caregiver were difficult. And like most parents in these situations, I faced the following:

- Fear of being separated from my baby (and as the years went by, my adolescent then young adult child) by death, for each year was treated as a blessed gift with little assurance that he would live another year
- Countless clinic appointments
- Countless surgeries
- Countless laboratory tests and procedures
- Countless medical emergency/ambulance runs
- Countless ancillary care services

- Navigating child social services and family care systems
- Burgeoning medication management protocols
- Wound sterilization and care
- Hours upon hours at the dialysis clinics
- Two kidney transplants and home dialysis
- Countless and lengthy all day and overnight stays on the hospital inpatient wards. I made a decision very early on that my child would not be separated from me for any length of time. I determined to be with him through the frightening and painful procedures; and if God said so, on the day or night that my child transitioned to heaven.
- Major strain on, and disillusionment about, my marriage
- Several financial wipeouts, including the loss of two homes due the catastrophic medical cost

Regarding my other children; a foster-adopted daughter with her early childhood losses and an older son who was as healthy as a horse, I tried to follow my father's example and be very careful to under promise and over deliver.

I was determined and worked hard to minimize disappointments and turn every possible upset or shift in plans into an adventure so that my children experienced their childhood/growing up as stable, safe, loving and enjoyable. This for my part required exceptional levels of planning and organization. This was exhausting yet quite satisfying when accomplished.

Caring for spouses

There are millions of devout men and women caring for spouses struggling and or suffering with physical, emotional or mental illnesses. In every case, the caretaker has the compounded responsibilities and multiple demands of family, home, and work.

My father and my mother

I know that this chapter repeats some information I've already said about my father elsewhere in this book. This is intentional as I wish to show him in a different context to make a point about the complex responsibilities of family caregivers. Here, my father's challenges and his loving determination to step up to the plate and stay the course is representative of a great many men and women.

Many credit women with the talent for multi-tasking. However, in my life it was my father who was able to work full time, manage his own business, care for three daughters while never missing a school visit, recital, concert or important life event, and care for my sick mother.

Now, my mother was not chronically ill, but she was occasionally bedbound due to a blood circulatory disorder. The condition ultimately resulted in a massive cerebral hemorrhage, which killed my mother when she was only 39. Before my mother's death, and even more so afterwards, my father did most of the cooking and cleaning until my sister and I were old enough to help out. He laundered and ironed our clothes and got us ready for school and church without fail. He helped us with our homework and did our hair most of the time (with the help of my aunt who was a beautician who gave us curls and bangs for special occasions like Christmas and Easter pageants, fashion shows, and concerts).

During my mother's bed rest time, my father made sure she was well fed, hydrated, and attended to her hygiene. He also scheduled and monitored her doctor's house calls and her medications. And he did all the shopping for groceries and clothing.

He did all of this while working nights full time at the railroad and running a commercial art business. He had homemaker services come in once or twice a week to help out with my sisters and I primarily for supervision so that he could run errands and manage his sign painting business. He came in early to put dinner on the table and check homework assignments, all before getting between three and four hours of sleep before waking up to go to work at the railroad.

My father was further challenged well into his senior years when my two younger sisters (then adults) fell prey to life-altering diseases. My middle sister had multiple sclerosis, and my younger sister, a chemical illness. His roles as family caregiver exceeded his life.

My father had a saying: "If a situation is not working out, make it work." He also told his daughters that, "The sky is your only limit." He lived by these sayings and demonstrated great possibilities in every endeavor. He always exuded faith in God, amazing energy, enthusiasm, laughter, and loving kindness to us because he never wanted us to feel like we were a burden to him.

When I was an adult, my father was my best friend, and we talked a lot about earlier years. It was only then that I realized how exhausted he had been much of the time while raising us. I feel that he had been able to push through relying on love, which I know can function just like adrenaline.

Sadly, at age 66 and less than one year after his retirement from the railroad, my father died from a heart attack. It was much too early.

He was never a drinker and he walked everywhere because he chose to never purchase or drive a car: one glance at him would tell you that he was a fit man. The sad truth was, my remarkable father was worn out. He gave all that he had as a family caregiver, but he did not create sufficient time for his own self-care.

A FEW RECOMMENDATIONS FOR FAMILY CAREGIVERS

Of course, I hope you follow the recommendations already presented in this book to prevent and treat compassion fatigue. But for you who are family caregivers, here are a few more key recommendations for your unique and challenging situation:

1. **Always prioritize your physical needs**: get good quality sleep—including an afternoon nap when possible—get good nutrition, have frequent medical checkups, exercise regularly, and get professional help when you experience depression.
2. **Avoid negativity, whether people-imposed or self-imposed:** try to connect with friends who immerse you in laughter and fun and who appreciate life.
3. **Ask for help**: make a list of things you have to do then recruit and delegate tasks wherever possible. Use outside agencies, faith-based organizations, and community and social clubs to help you do this.
4. **Research community resources:** learn about and utilize caregiver support groups, home health aides or homemakers, and volunteers from your local churches.
5. **Develop your own therapeutic community**: these are people to help you cope with and voice your feelings. Choose people who will easily shift your thoughts to more positive thinking.

6. **Take breaks and relax frequently**: steal moments for yourself during early mornings, late evenings, or when your loved one is napping.
7. **Make to-do lists daily**: do this to stay organized and to determine the order of importance.
8. **Just say no:** say no to other people and outside obligations when you are stretched thin and tired.
9. **Have fun diversions**: take along fun activities to engage in when waiting during long appointments. These could be knitting, crochet, a sketch pad, Sudoku, or crossword puzzle books, a great novel, and MP3s with soothing, uplifting music.

SOME PARTING THOUGHTS

The scenarios I have shared in this chapter are just a small representation of the many types of scenarios faced by millions of family caregivers. So it is with the deepest respect I acknowledge every type of situation and especially you, the compassionate and responsible people who step up to the plate. I sincerely hope that you are blessed with a supportive community to help you as you help your family members in need. It is my prayer that you attend also with great diligence to your own wellbeing as you travel along this uphill journey.

CONTACT THE CAREGIVER HOTLINE

Should you ever feel overwhelmed or unable to deal with the demands of being a family caregiver, there is a hotline you can call where you will find a listening ear and, when you ask for it, needed advice.

Caregiver Hotline
1-877-333-5885
Mon-Fri: 7 am – 11 pm ET
Sat: 9 am – 5 pm ET

CHAPTER 14:
A FEW FINAL THOUGHTS

For those of you who struggle with guilt regarding self-care, answer this question: What greater gift can you give to those you love than your own wholeness?

—Shannon Tanner,
Worthy: The POWER of Wholeness

THIS BOOK IS MY GIFT TO YOU

I wrote this book to help you, you who daily engage in difficult situations, situations that most others would avoid. Many of you run towards danger to rescue others. You extend your hands to stem the flow of blood and save the life force, when many would not be able to even look in that direction. You keep your eyes, your thoughts, and your compassion focused on the needs, safety, and wellbeing of the suffering, the victimized, and the traumatized. Many in society are unaware of those who suffer, or they pretend that these needs do not exist. For most people, caregiving is simply not their calling. But you know, and you see, and you have committed your love, energies, and skills to serving those in need. This book is my gift to you, for you are truly heroes.

My gift is to help do what is also in your best interest and know that you have the power to restore and maintain your own health and wellbeing throughout your years of dedicated and compassionate service to others.

PRESERVING COMPASSION SATISFACTION

As a service worker and caregiver, you sacrifice much, but you can also experience a great deal of satisfaction from the very important work you do. The term for the satisfaction and joy often experienced by those in helping professions is called compassion satisfaction (Stamm, 2002). Compassion satisfaction is the feeling of competence that you get because you helped someone and made a difference in their lives. As helping professionals, you are always making a difference, and I hope you often feel satisfaction because of your compassion, which motivates you to do the work you do.

But compassion satisfaction can be greatly diminished or even lost when we fail to preserve it via diligent self-care habits. We need to work as individuals, as teams, and as organizations to restore and maintain it.

A MESSAGE TO MANAGERS

And now I'd like to say something to the managers who have read this book.

In this book, I have tried to identify the benefits of intentional self-care practices, and I hope that this book helps you promote a work environment where all staff are aware of their vulnerability to secondary and vicarious trauma and where they practice adequate self-care in order to promote employee effectiveness, job retention, and satisfaction. I have also provided practical suggestions to help staff bounce back in the face of overwhelming and emotionally intense demands.

Work settings have a profound effect on a professional's vulnerability to secondary and vicarious trauma as you and your staff often find yourself in contentious situations, including risks to your personal safety. And of course, diminishing resources and an overtaxed or diminishing workforce can worsen the traumatic stress syndrome for a work team. No one expects this dynamic to change for the better any time soon, if ever.

But sadly, too few of you and too few of your workers get the opportunity to process, verbalize, and understand the secondary (and at times direct) trauma that you experience as part of your work. Because of this, it is difficult to recognize and address the early warning signs of traumatic stress overload in yourselves, your colleagues, and those who work for you.

On top of this, organizations actually increase the risk of vicarious trauma for their staff when they do not provide respite. Indeed, the respite they provide should include shared coverage, adequate time off, realistic caseloads, qualified supervision, acknowledging the severity and pervasiveness of the client's traumatic experiences, training for staff to identify and address signs of traumatic stress, continuing education, and sufficient vacation time and personal psychotherapy opportunities (Saakvitne and Pearlman, 1996).

Might I suggest that you, as managers, need to train new staff on the subject of compassion fatigue, aka secondary and vicarious traumatic stress. Doing this will help new staff avoid compassion fatigue and will help you keep valued staff safe, effective, and energized in their work. This training will also help your staff to self-regulate during and after intensely stressful events.

And last, but certainly not least, don't forget to attend to your own self-care with the same diligence that you attend to your staff's self-care. In the end, remember to be authentic with what you offer and be realistic about what you can do. And remember to encourage your staff, because a kind supportive word can go a long way when resources run out.

A MESSAGE TO CLERGY (PASTORS, MINISTRY LEADERS, AND OTHER SPIRITUAL LEADERS)

I offer a brief word to my Elders, brothers and sisters in the clergy. Because as part of a pastoral family I observed you in action during my youth, and I served alongside some of you over the course of much of my adult life, I have received this insight and revelation. Neither Saturday nor Sunday is a day of rest for you. For on these days you are fully engaged in the ministry service. I humbly urge you to pick another day when you and your families are truly resting. Discharging and recharging; healing your spirits, minds and bodies; laughing/refreshing. Given the vast complexities of serving in the mission and ministry, family sacrifice is a natural part of the call to serve. However, when you try to manage all elements of godly service on your own; when you try to be completely available for all of the needs of both your membership and your staff, self-neglect is absolutely unavoidable. The consequences to your physical, psychological and emotional health are significant and potentially quite detrimental. In far too many cases exhausting oneself in this way leaves little or nothing left to give when you return home to love one's who are waiting to see you, share with you, and love you. Subsequently, family disillusionment is the highly probable outcome. I could share lots of stories about my aunts and uncles a.k.a. the preacher's kids. Many areas of their lives were in stark opposition to my grandparents. So many aspects served as a painful disappointment yet the contribution to those disappointments were shared by all because as leaders my Pastoral Grands' were not great delegator's of duties and tasks that could have afforded them more time with their children and spouses and for self-care.

Additionally, this level of physical and emotional drain can to some significant degree fracture your faith. Continuous bombardment and absorption of distressing and sometimes traumatic content that plagues the human condition has been known to cause too many of you to heartbreakingly question your faith. It is imperative that while protecting confidentiality, you seek ways to professionally process and discharge some of this disturbing content to save and preserve your vessel; which is your spirit, mind and body.

While working on various ministries during the week I observed Pastors and often their families in the church building with seemingly very little home life. They may have been as I was, under the influence drawn again from my own family, operating under the impression that because I was doing Godly service, I would be alright. I was wrong. God commanded us to take a day of rest each and every week. Also to move away from the people periodically for time alone; silence, refreshing and most important to hear His voice. Disobeying this command had dire; near fatal consequences for me. This does not have to be the case for you. As you embrace this discipline of self-care for yourself please also impart it's practice as a mandate firmly to your ministry leaders.

Countless numbers of your flock are needy people; very needy people who draw continuously on your inner resources. Not being consciously aware, you allow them to drain you. Some call this burnout. Others call it drain out. There is a tendency to try to personally address every need; certainly out of love, compassion and a strong sense of responsibility, AND perhaps at times, your own need to be needed. Combine this with your leadership and management duties; and include all of the interesting personalities of your staff ….you are like war time soldiers badly in need of R and R.

Why?... because you do not "count the cost" to your spirit, mind and body.

Remember the many biblical stories about the temples built for God. Remember also how these sacred edifices would be cared for; preserved and nurtured. It is our belief that our body-minds are the temples of God. And so likewise, nurture and preserve yourselves with all diligence, intent and Godly love.

A MESSAGE TO SOCIETY: HELP ME HELP THE HELPERS

When our society supports those who support and protect the suffering, the victimized, and the traumatized, we break the cycle of pain and disruption for society's vulnerable and mitigate the negative effects that tragedy has had on their lives.

As a society, we must support and strengthen those who have diligently trained and dedicated their lives to preventing abuse and tragedy and to helping out in its wake. In addition to often risking their own safety, these helpers risk suffering with compassion fatigue, to make a difference in the lives of the most vulnerable members of our society.

However, in communities across America, staff and resources have been drastically reduced at a time when they are needed more than ever. One example of this is the shrinking resources that child welfare workforces have been experiencing, causing much higher caseloads, which in turn leads to emotional exhaustion of workers, increased staff turnover, and lower service quality for children. The average caseload for child welfare workers is now between 24 and 31 children. All too frequently the numbers can be as many 100 children per worker, all while the Child Welfare League of America suggests a caseload ratio of 12 to 15. Similar scenarios plague each of the human services systems and weigh heavily on the individual helper.

In case you needed more proof of this, here are just a few statistics to illustrate this concern: 14% of all men imprisoned in the United States were abused children, 36% of all women in prison were abused children; 59% of abused children will likely be arrested as a juvenile, 28% more will likely to be arrested as an adult, and 30% will be more likely to commit a violent crime. As many as two thirds of the people in treatment for drug abuse reported abuse and neglect in their childhood. This does not have to be the case when we as a society help the remarkable people who are helping our children.

A FINAL WORD OF COUNSEL ABOUT SELF-CARE

The harvest truly is great, but the laborers are few. –Luke 10:2

As a service worker, you have a lot of responsibility, authority, and influence as you care for those in need. Your role requires a lot of patience, planning, skill, training, and expertise. You interact with people who are very difficult, desperate, depressed, fearful, terrified, hurt, broken, and angry. Your service is impacted by major pressures, staff shortages, multiple disappointments, detrimental lengths of days, and very limited resources.

At the same time, client numbers and needs are burgeoning. And on top of all that, society often misunderstands and underestimates the work that you do. All of this, along with your own personal life stresses, can lead to potentially debilitating daily choices that can fracture your spirit. Yet you care very deeply because you know that you are very much needed, and so against all odds, you work through your fatigue and emotional distress to meet the needs of others.

For these reasons, I urge you never to forget your own self-care. Make choices daily that include you and that make your health and wellbeing a top priority. And watch for the signs, both subtle and not-so-subtle, that you need to step back and breathe, release, recover, and recharge. Remember to be good to yourself.

There are not enough of us available to rescue, counsel, treat, or care for the victims of trauma: the number of helping professionals who enter the field and then leave is staggering. They leave because they are physically and emotionally worn out, frustrated, burned out, exhausted, and sick. Those who remain are stretched beyond human capacity to meet the continuing and relentless work demands. This too does not have to be the case. Caring and compassionate service providers can be retained and remain healthy and satisfied with their jobs when they are able to understand and intentionally prevent compassionate fatigue from happening to them. This takes education, guidance, and support from all key players in this service to humankind.

Paint brushes

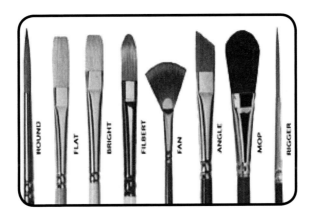

I love to tell this story at the end of the most of my speaking engagements. It is a real story; however, I did not realize its importance to my life until recently. Rather, the revelations embedded in this story came long after my physical and emotional collapse. Wherever you are in your stage of development in the work, I pray this story is meaningful for you.

My mother had fragile health during my early years, and tragically, she died leaving behind three little girls, whom my father finished raising on his own. My father had to take us with him most everywhere while he was supervising and caring for us. He worked nights as a porter for the railroad, and during the day he dropped us off and picked us up from school. My father was also an entrepreneurial commercial artist, and so very often he was in his studio, which was on the top floor of a very large church building, stretching very huge canvases and then painting in the lettering.

He often took us with him to the studio, which was large enough to ride our bicycles, jump rope, and play jacks, and most importantly, to sit and do our homework and study while he worked. He also taught my sisters Denise, Jeri and I how to sing a cappella in this studio. My father was also an Opera Singer.

One special feature about these particular outings was that daddy would allow us to help him do the lined layout for his signs. After carefully marking in his measurements, my sister Denise and I would stand on opposite ends of this huge rectangular sign and hold the charcoal strings in perfect position. Once he was satisfied that the string was in the right place, my father would snap the string and perfect lines would appear across the sign, which was always several yards wide.

Later, after daddy had painted in his perfectly-proportioned letters, he would clean his paint brushes, which was an even more fascinating process. We would watch him dip them in turpentine and wipe them off over and over until every speck of paint was removed from the bristles and the handle of the brush. Next, using this soft doeskin cloth, he would dip the fine sable hairs of the brushes repeatedly in a linseed oil and then stroke the hairs and handles ever so lovingly. Finally, he would gently place each brush in its own slot in a velvet-lined case.

My sister and I would stare at this process in wonder, forever trying to understand why he spent so much time on it. And as children will, we loved to ask him "Why?" so that he could tell us the story, which he did, over and over again. He said, "Baby, my artistic talent is a gift from God. And in appreciation to Him, I give my gift to help others; however, I would not be able to share and give my gift if I do not take excellent care of the tools of my gift. And those tools are these brushes. And that is why I take such great time and care of them."

The revelation in this story is this: the gift that you have, and the gift that you give to the people we serve is your caring and compassion. You give your commitment, time, efforts, determination, presence, listening, patience, gentleness, respect, forgiveness, acts of kindness, and love to humanity. And the tools of your gift are your mind, body, and spirit. I lovingly ask you to treat each of these mindfully with tenderness, care, and love. Find a sacred resting place for your mind, body, and spirit to restore, refresh, and recharge. As much as you give compassion to those in need, I pray you diligently attend to self-compassion. After all, you are the very hands of God.

HOW YOU CAN HELP ME HELP YOU

Writing a book is no easy task. And perhaps, neither is reading one. I have given you a lot of information in this book, which contains my accumulated knowledge, experience, and perhaps even a little wisdom. And now, I would like you to do something for me.

Please assist me in connecting with the services systems listed above so that I can offer my services to them. Please spread the word of my intent to advance a healthy agency initiative that will potentially help the most helpers and touch the lives of millions across this country. If granted this opportunity, I will work with you to determine which areas of human services in your communities and/or your organization are most in need.

I would be grateful for the opportunity to talk with you more about compassion fatigue and how you can raise awareness and help others combat it. I also welcome the opportunity to provide you with more information about the work of The Kyer Group as well as to answer any questions.

Thank you, and God bless you as you serve others.

ABOUT THE AUTHOR

Beverly Kyer has a Master's Degree in Social Work and is a member of the Academy of Certified Social Workers. She has postgraduate certificates and over three decades of experience in integrated approach to readjustment counseling, post-traumatic stress disorder, social research for the mentally ill, and employee assistance program coordination. Beverly was also certified in Toronto Canada at the Traumatology Institute as a Compassion Fatigue Specialist.

Beverly became a Clinical Social Worker specializing in pediatric oncology; PTSD in Vietnam Veterans, and Psychiatric Day Hospital Treatment. She spent much of her career with the Veteran's Administration Veteran's Outreach Center and Medical Center in The Bronx, New York City. Beverly also spent more than a decade as a direct care service provider in the foster care system. She also spent seven years as an urban high school counselor, providing emotional and psychological support for students and staff.

Two episodes of heart failure led Beverly to make a major downshift in her life by resigning from full time employment, joining the self-employed, and devoting her life to help others who work in highly stressful environments. Beverly lectures around the country on compassion fatigue, which is sometimes known as secondary or vicarious traumatic stress.

Beverly has three grown children: two sons and an adopted daughter, and she lives in Northern California in a quiet cul-de-sac near the delta. Oil painting, music, movies, and good books are among her passions.

REFERENCES

American Psychiatric Association. (2000). Diagnostic and statistical manual of mental disorders (4th ed., text rev.). Washington, DC.

Bandura, A. (1977). Social learning theory. Englewood Cliffs, NJ: Prentice Hall.

Baranowski & Lauer, (2012); What is PTSD?: 3 Steps to Healing Trauma,

Beck, A. T. (1976). Cognitive therapy and emotional disorders. New York, NY: International Universities Press.

Burns, D. (1999). *Feeling good, the new mood therapy*. New York, NY: William Morrow and Co.

Erickson, C. A. (1989). Rape and the family. In C. R. Figley (1989). Treating stress in families, 257-290. NY: Brunner/Mazel.

Fendrich, M., Mackesy-Amiti, M.E., Wislar, J.S., & Goldstein, P.J. (1997). Childhood abuse and the use of inhalants: Differences by degree of use. *American Journal of Public Health,* 87(5):765-769.

Figley, C. R. (1995). *Compassion fatigue: Coping with secondary traumatic stress disorder in those who treat the traumatized.* New York, NY: Brunner-Mazel.

Figley, C. R. (Ed). (2002). *Treating compassion fatigue/psychosocial stress series.* New York, NY: Brunner-Routledge.

Goleman, Daniel Jay. (1995) *Emotional Intelligence*; Rando House Publishing

Harlow, C. W. (1999). Prior Abuse Reported by Inmates and Probationers, in Bureau of Justice Statistics Selected Findings, US Department of Justice. Retrieved from http://www.bjs.gov/content/pub/pdf/parip.pdf

Jacobson, E. (1934). *You must relax: A practical method of reducing the strains of modern living.* New York, NY: Whittlesey house, McGraw-Hill.

McCann, I.L., & Pearlman, L.A. (1990). Vicarious traumatization: A framework for understanding the psychological effects of working with victims. *Journal of Traumatic Stress, 3* (1),131-149.

Meichenbaum, D. H. (1975). A self instructional approach to stress management: A proposal for stress inoculation. In C. D. Spielberger and I Sarsason (Eds.), *Stress and Anxiety* (2). New York, NY: Wiley.

National Child Traumatic Stress Network. (2011). Secondary Traumatic Stress: A fact Sheet for Child-Serving Professionals.

Pearlman, L. A. & Saakvitne, K. W. (1996, 1995). National Association of Social Workers. Government Relations Update, Child Welfare Workforce.

Perry, B.D. (1998). Homeostasis, stress, trauma and adaptation. *Child and Adolescent Psychiatric Clinic of North America,* (7) 33-51.

Remer, R. & Elliot, J. (1988). Characteristics of secondary victims of sexual assault. International Journal of Family Psychiatry, 9:4, 373-387.

Social Work Policy Institute. (2010, January). Research to practice brief.

Stamm, B.H. (1995). *Secondary traumatic stress: self-care issues for clinicians, researchers, and educators.* Brooklandville, MD: Sidran Press.

Stamm, B.H. (1997). Work-related secondary traumatic stress. *PTSD Research Quarterly*, 5 (2) 1-6.

Stamm, B.H. (2002). Measuring compassion satisfaction as well as fatigue: Developmental history of the compassion fatigue and satisfaction test. In C.R. Figley (Ed.), 107-119.

Stamm, B.H. & Figley, C.R. (2009, November) Advances in the Theory of Compassion Satisfaction and Fatigue and its Measurement with the ProQOL 5. Measuring compassion satisfaction as well as fatigue: Developmental history of the compassion satisfaction and fatigue test. Pocatello, ID: ProQOL.org.

Stamm, B.H. (2010). *The concise proqol manual, 2nd ed.* Pocatello, ID: ProQOL.org.

Taylor, S. (1998) *Health Psychology, 2nd ed.* New York, NY: McGraw-Hill.

U.S. Department of Health and Human Services, Administration on Children, Youth, and Families. Child Maltreatment (2008). Washington, DC: Government Printing Office. Retrieved from http://www.acf.hhs.gov/programs/cb/pubs/cm08/summary.htm

U.S. Department of Health and Human Services, Administration for Children and Families, Children's Bureau. (2011). Child Maltreatment 2010. Retrieved from http://www.acf.hhs.gov/programs/cb/stats_research/index.htm#can

Verbosky, S. J. & Ryan, D. A. (1988). Female partners of Vietnam veterans: Stress by proximity. Issues in Mental Health NurWsing. 9:1, 95–104.

White, P. N. & Rollins, J. C. (1981). Rape: A family crisis. Family Relations, 30 (1), 103-109.

Widom, C. S. & Maxfield, M. G. (2001). An Update on the Cycle of Violence, Research in Brief, Washington, DC: U.S. Department of Justice, National Institute of Justice, NCJ 184894

Wikipedia. (2015). Compassion fatigue. Retrieved from http://en.wikipedia.org/w/index. php?title=Compassion_fatigue&oldid=639625141